JUN **1 3** 2005

3-12-12(6)
32744(12)

Tai Chi

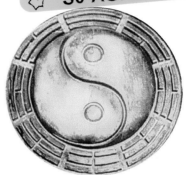

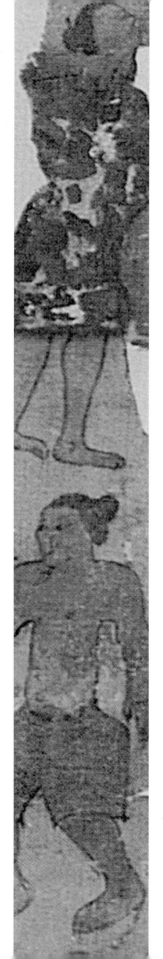

THE SIMPLE ART OF
Tai Chi

Qu Lei Lei

**Foreword by
Grand Master Chen Xiao Wang**

STERLING PUBLISHING CO., INC.
NEW YORK

Library of Congress Cataloging-in-Publication
Data available

10 9 8 7 6 5 4 3 2 1

Published in 2004 by Sterling Publishing Co., Inc.
387 Park Avenue South, New York, NY 10016

First published in Great Britain in 2004 by Cico Books
32 Great Sutton Street London EC1V 0NB
© 2004 Cico Books
Text © 2004 Qu Lei Lei

Distributed in Canada by Sterling Publishing
c/o Canadian Manda Group,
165 Dufferin Street, Toronto, Ontario,
Canada M6K 3H6

Edited by Robin Gurdon
Photographs by Geoff Dann
Design by Paul Wood

Printed and bound in Singapore

ISBN 1-4027-1651-6

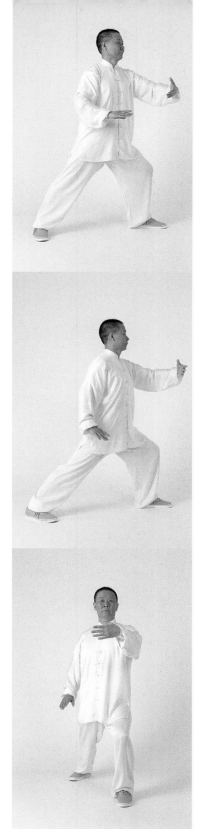

Contents

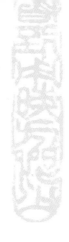

Foreword

Chen Wang Ting (1600–1680), the titan of *Tai Chi Quan*, based on the ancient Chinese philosophy of *yin* and *yang*, combined the theories of Chinese medicine with martial art actions into one—combining philosophy, *Tai Chi,* with *Quan*, meaning "fist." In the past it was more widely used on the battlefield, but nowadays it is almost exclusively practiced for keeping fit, evolving into different styles—such as *yang*, *wu*, *sun*, and *woo*—each with many different forms—including the 24 shown in this book which were produced originally by China's Central Sports Committee. Even though the many styles and forms are different, the basic philosophy always remains the same.

When learning and practicing *Tai Chi Quan* for keeping fit, it is important to always follow the rules, enabling the body's circulation system to flourish, and to avoid, as well as treat, illness. The study and practice of its philosophy can improve mental health and keep the mind balanced. As mental health always influences physical health and physical health likewise affects the mind *Tai Chi* cultivates both mental and physical health. Thousands and thousands of Chinese people have recovered and been healed from many complicated problems through *Tai Chi* exercise. Their health and longevity have been increased, and so too their moral standards.

Tai Chi's history as a practical martial art emphasizes the importance of centering yourself firmly and keeping stable at all times. Any reaction depends on the direction, angle, and speed of an attack. Good balance lets you control your own natural movements, giving you the opportunity to stretch or deflect an attack, and retaliate into your opponent's "empty," weak point. This is the central theory of *Tai Chi Quan* as a martial art: the body should never lean away from the center and always be able to push out with force in all directions. All the actions of the Forms are designed as responses to an enemy's attack from the front, side, or back. Whatever the movement or new situation, always keep the *dan tian*—the central, pivoting point in the middle of your body—at the center of your movements, linking all other body movements together by "gathering thousands of ways in one."

Tai Chi is ideal for keeping fit and as a martial art. However, there are always those who pass on mistakes, misleading the learner, which is a waste of time. Even worse, some practice *Tai Chi* against its original philosophy. Therefore, when you start to learn *Tai Chi* you must have a clear understanding of its aims and theory. Only then will you be able to improve step by step until you reach the highest state.

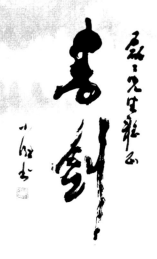

Grand Master Chen Xiao Wang

May, 2004, Switzerland

Calligraphy dedicated to Mr. Qu Lei Lei by Grand Master Chen Xiao Wang

Introduction

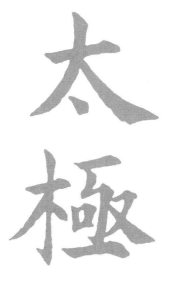

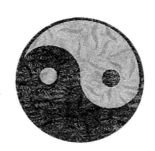

What are *Tai Chi* and *Yin Yang*?

Tai Chi and *yin yang*, also called the *Tao*, are central concepts in Chinese philosophy, and together they provide a key that can open the door to mind–body harmony. Through observation and research of everything in the universe, ancient Chinese philosophers concluded that there is a basic, regular construction common to all phenomena, from the entire cosmos to a single piece of dust. The *tai chi* pattern, interlocking black (*yin*) and white (*yang*) shapes, make up the *yin yang* symbol—a visual representation of the philosophy of the *Tao*. The symbol has four basic messages.

First, through the use of black and white, the symbol describes the basic relationship between all things. That is, that every object and every concept must have an opposite, and that one cannot exist without the other. For example, sky is *yang* while earth is *yin*; light is *yang*, shadow *yin*. This applies equally to man and woman, fire and water, dragon and tiger, heart and kidney, top and bottom, outside and inside, hot and cold, movement and stillness, body and spirit.

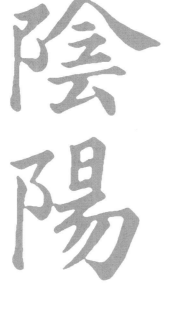

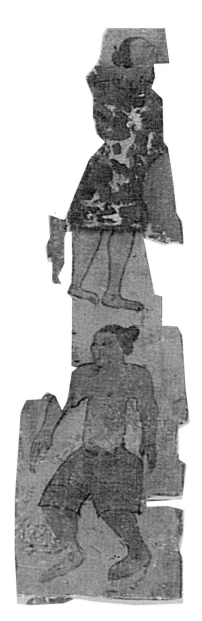

Second, the symbol shows how *yin* and *yang* are constantly moving to maintain universal balance and stability: When one part of the pattern is finishing, the other has already begun. The result is a perfect circle.

Third, we learn that *yin* and *yang* always include an element of their opposite: There is always *yin* within *yang* and *yang* within *yin*, as shown by the two round dots of the opposite color in the pattern. During their movement *yin* and *yang* are always changing and transferring to each other. In life, this manifests in, for example, the concepts of day and night, spring planting and autumn harvesting, and man and woman.

Finally, through their movement and transferral, *yin* and *yang* each expand through the circle of five elements (the *wu xing*—water, wood, fire, metal and earth) and the *bagua* (the Eight Diagrams; see caption, page 13) until all things in the universe are made from *yin* and *yang*.

Above and right:
Painted in around the second century BC, these figures are among the earliest representation of *Dao Yin* exercises, a forerunner to *Tai Chi*.

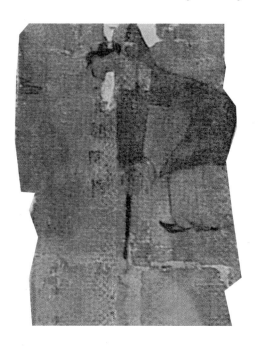

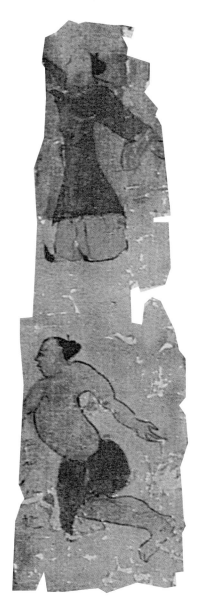

Above:
These figures (also from paintings dating from the second century BC) show clearly the similarities bewteen the stretching movements of *Dao Yin* and the later *Tai Chi*.

Chi

The Chinese word *chi* can be directly translated into English as "air," but in *Tai Chi, Chi Gong,* and traditional Chinese medicine, the word has a far broader and significant meaning. The way in which we breathe and move and the efficiency of our circulation and digestive systems show the quality of our life and our spiritual condition, or *chi.* For example, someone who is happy and energetic has strong *chi;* while someone suffering from depression or lethargy has weak *chi.* When *chi* is strong we are healthy; when it is weak we are unwell. Some people try to make *chi* a mysterious or superstitious concept, but it is simply a measure of health.

Tai Chi combines breathing, improved circulation, and muscle movement, as well as the body's spirit, in a single exercise system which aims to enhance *chi* and so our mental and physical well-being.

The force of *chi* does not only affect living forms. The Chinese believe in the *chi* of sky (including the weather) and the *chi* of earth. These are important because the six different life forms known to us—human, animal, bird, fish, insect, and plant—are all born from the overall life forms, the sky and the earth. The Chinese believe that when the sky and earth move together, or "make love"—using air, light, and water represented by thunder, lightning, and rain—all other life is made possible.

Since ancient times, practitioners of Taoist exercises put themselves directly between the sky and the earth when performing their routines. Forming a link between the forces of nature, especially during gales and storms, a practitioner felt able to absorb maximum *chi* from the sky and the earth, increasing his or her energy levels and overall well-being. In Taoist philosophy, this is called *Tian Ren He Yi*—the combination of humans and nature.

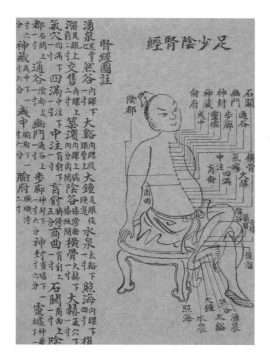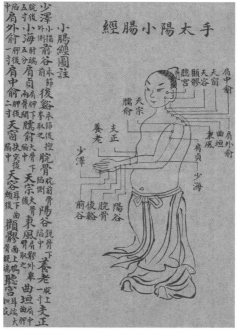

Above:
Chi is believed to flow through meridians, special energy channels in the body. Medical scrolls from the tenth century show the development of the concept of meridians.

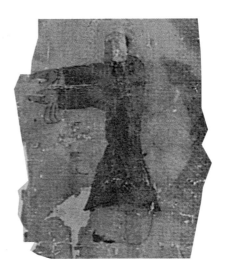

Chi Gong and *Tai Chi Quan*

At least 3,000 years ago, China already had formal exercise systems aimed at treating illness, keeping the body fit, and securing a long life. In the Spring–Autumn Period (770–476BC) of the Zhou dynasty there are detailed records about *Xing Qi* (literally, "the movement of the *chi*"), *Tu Na* (a way of breathing, literally meaning "in and out"), and, during the Han dynasty (206BC–AD220), *Dao Yin* (the precursor to *Tai Chi* and literally meaning "guide lead"). All present similar exercises that show the correct way to breathe to allow the free-flow of *chi* through the body, and the correct way to combine breathing and movement to stabilize the whole body-system. These are the earliest *Chi Gong*, or formulated keep-fit exercises, developed in China.

Hua Tuo, the famous doctor of the Han dynasty, then combined these early exercise systems with movements he observed in animals, to create a series of exercises called *Wu Qin Xi* (the "Five Animals' Game"), based on the tiger, deer, bear, monkey, and bird. After the Sui dynasty (581–618), those exercises developed

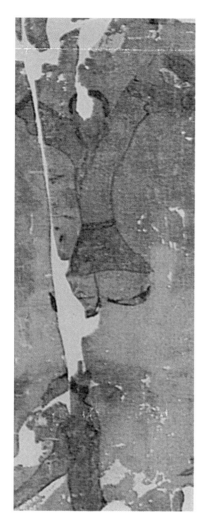

into more stylized *Chi Gong* forms such as *Ba Duan Jin* ("Eight Pieces of Silk"), *Shi Er Duan Jin* ("Twelve Pieces of Silk"), and *Yi Jin Jing*.

At the end of the Ming dynasty (1368–1644), using Taoist philosophy as a base, *Chi Gong* was combined with features of existing martial arts to create *Tai Chi Quan*, which we normally abbreviate to *Tai Chi*. This new exercise system gave people a means of keeping fit as well as a form of self-defence; it improved participants' moral and spiritual focus; and *Tai Chi* offered such low-impact exercise, that it proved suitable for practice among all age groups and levels of fitness. And it could be practiced anywhere. As a result, nowadays, all over the world, more and more people are participating in *Tai Chi*.

Tai Chi has five major styles—*Chen, Yang, Wu, Woo,* and *Sun*—each of which has many different sub-styles and Forms. However, the basic philosophy for practice and exercise are the same. In this book we introduce the 24 Forms of the most popular *Yang* style, which was designed by China's top masters in the 1950s. It is a clear and relatively short set of exercises, including most of the fundamental features of the philosophy of *Tai Chi*, making it the ideal starting point for beginners.

Above and opposite:
Dao Yin exercise focused on combining the breath with movement, just as *Tai Chi* would in the centuries to follow.

Right:
This *yin yang* symbol is cast in gold and surrounded by the Eight Diagrams (eight sets of three lines—some broken, some unbroken) of the *bagua*. In Chinese divination, the Eight Diagrams were used to represent the elemental forces.

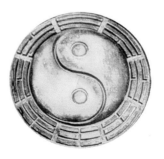

Key Points

The Important Aspects of *Tai Chi* Exercises

Although *Tai Chi* is a martial art, it does not rely upon the strength of the body, but on the power of the mind. This means that you can utilize the Forms as an exercise regime no matter what your state of health or fitness. (However, if you are unsure about whether or not *Tai Chi* is suitable for you, consult your doctor or medical practitioner before beginning.) When first learning the art of *Tai Chi* you might feel you are spending a lot of time practicing and remembering each movement—but don't worry, you will get there. Little by little the movements will become natural and you can go into the exercises in more depth. As *Tai Chi* is a philosophical art as well as a means of fitness, you should always take into account the eight key concepts described in this chapter—whether you are a beginner or a master—to ensure that you gain the most benefit from your practice.

Stay upright, weight balanced—stand stable as a pine

The most important point is to keep your mind sincere and uncluttered during your practice, thus helping to give your body perfect stillness. You should always feel rooted to the ground, even when moving. Never start a movement when you feel even slightly unbalanced. Before beginning, stay still and balance yourself. Then, however complex the movement, you will stay stable as a mountain and proud as the pine, whatever forces of nature are thrown against your practice.

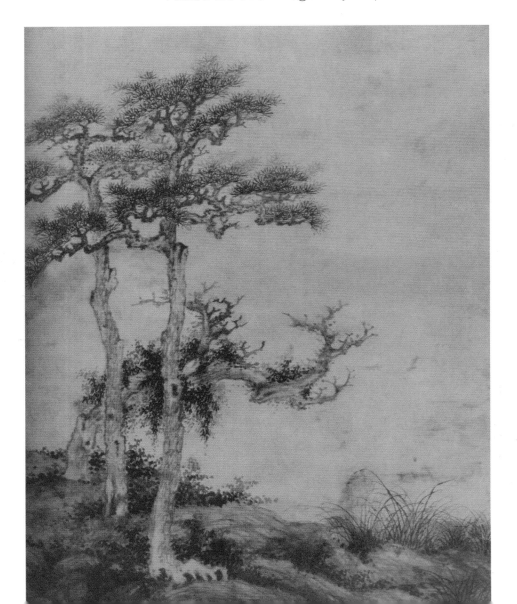

Keep the body relaxed and tender with no tension or forced strength—walking like a cat

Let your whole body be relaxed and soft—like a leopard hunting. During *Tai Chi*, it is vital to be relaxed, so never force energy through your muscles. Don't mistake this softness for a lack of effort. During each movement, consciously relax the muscles and joints that you are not actively using. Always push your weight downward, letting the *chi* flow upward. Observe a cat walking—it moves softly and quietly, but is always ready to pounce.

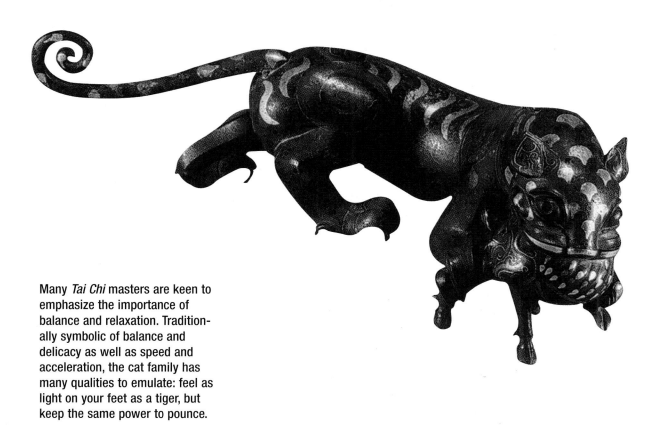

Many *Tai Chi* masters are keen to emphasize the importance of balance and relaxation. Traditionally symbolic of balance and delicacy as well as speed and acceleration, the cat family has many qualities to emulate: feel as light on your feet as a tiger, but keep the same power to pounce.

Move smoothly and naturally, never be jerky—as a floating cloud and flowing water

From the moment you start moving during *Tai Chi* there is never a time when any part of the body is completely still. Use your mind rather than your physical strength to progress smoothly and naturally from phase to phase. The movements require only a natural, circular progression, free from sharp jolts. Lao Tzu, the attributed founder of Taoist philosophy, said, "The most prized characteristics are those of water." Water flows around stones and all other obstacles, quietly but continuously searching for a path, until eventually it reaches the sea.

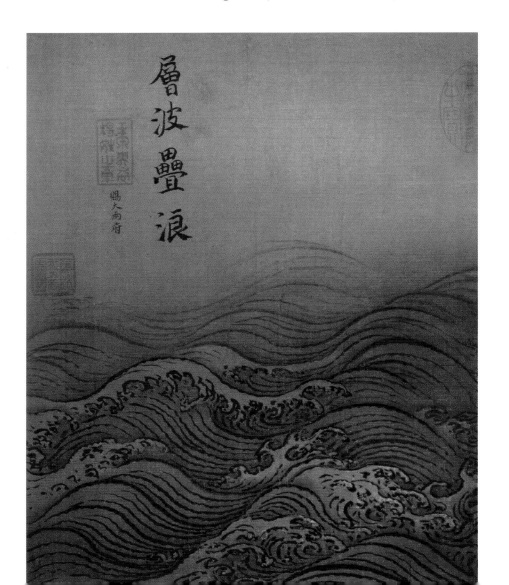

Coordinate your whole body as one, relating all parts to one another—as the cogs of a watch

When one part of your body moves, all parts move. This fundamental feature of *Tai Chi* ensures that every part of the body is coordinated during exercise. Beginners may forget one part when concentrating on another, or may not quite coordinate their movements. At first, learn each element of a movement separately before joining them together, just as you would learn each hand separately when attempting to play a new piece on the piano. Whenever the arm or torso moves, it always follows the *dan tian* (the central point of balance located just below the navel) and is led by the waist. An action is never led by a push or pull of the arms or legs—the waist moves and the limbs always follow. Understanding this allows every part of the body to become better coordinated.

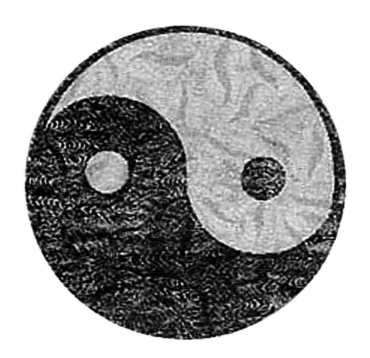

Distinguish between solidness and emptiness, hardness and softness—as the change in the four seasons

Once you have learned the structure of the Forms, you can focus on the contrast between solidness and emptiness, hardness and softness in your body. During the Forms, your weight is always shifting as you move continuously between attack and defence positions. Always be clear when and where your energy is being used—which parts are relaxed and which are working; which are solid with weight and which are empty; and also which parts of the body are moving and turning.

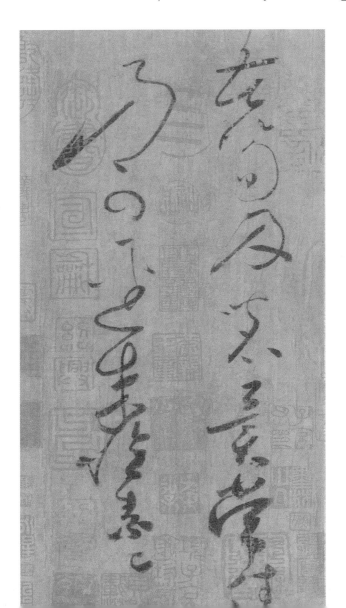

Concentrate the mind, let your spirit lead your movement— the body must follow the *chi*

The procession of *Tai Chi* exercise requires the body's movement to be led by the mind, so that spirit is placed into every part of the exercise. First, relax the body and empty the mind, breathing naturally. Second, concentrate the mind on the *dan tian* (see pages 19 and 30), so that you can call upon its balance through all the movements.

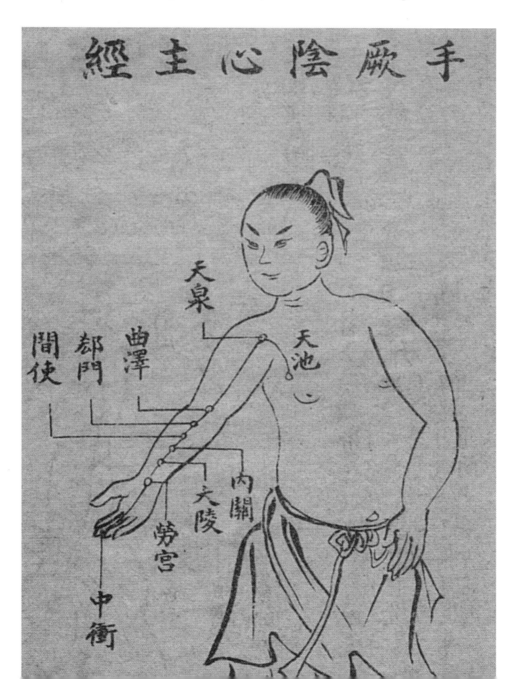

Breathe naturally, combining the breath with every movement—as the ocean's tides ebb and flow

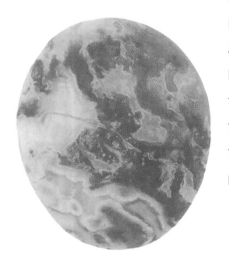

Breathing is very important in *Tai Chi* exercise. Avoid fast, irregular, or shallow breathing, and never hold your breath. Breathing must be natural, slow, deep, and smooth—just as the sea's tides ebb and flow. Generally, prepare to begin each Form by breathing in, and, as you complete the movements, breathe out. Usually let your breathing follow your body: if you are bringing your body in during the Form, breathe in. When moving outward, kicking, or punching, breathe out.

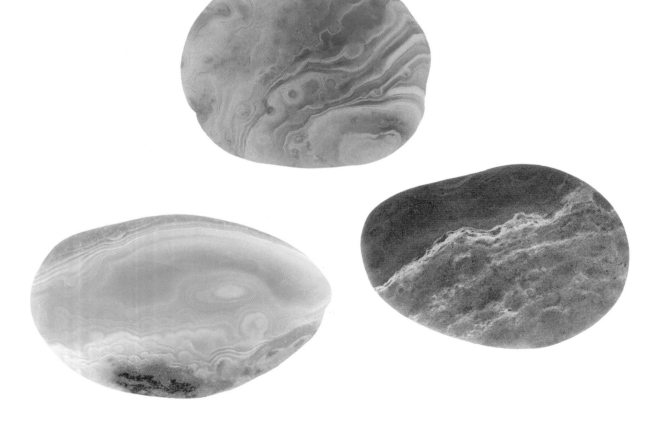

Follow the rules, progress gradually, and never give up— enjoy your healthy and long life

Do not try to rush to success. Instead, learn the Forms bit by bit, movement by movement, until each is correct, with the body, mind, and breathing in unison. Gradually improve the quality of each movement. The 24 Forms in this book include most of the important movements and all the key points of *Tai Chi* philosophy, which, when learned properly, will allow you to switch easily to other styles of *Tai Chi*. Try to avoid irregular exercise: enjoy working on your *Tai Chi* practice for a little time every day. You will experience both physical and mental long-term benefits—and, just like the Chinese saying, "You will have the longevity of a mountain."

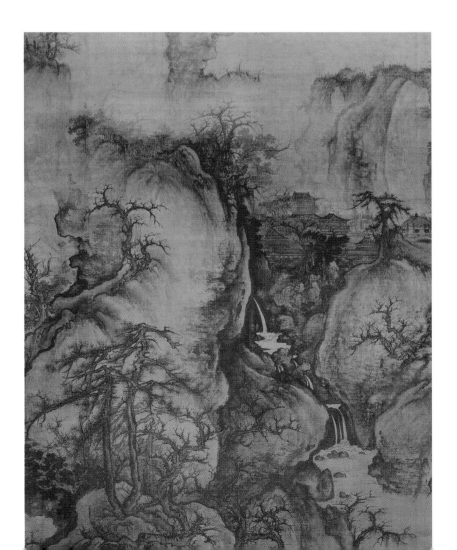

Basic Techniques

Before you can fully practice the 24 Forms of *Tai Chi* covered in this book, you will need to master a selection of basic techniques. As a form of exercise, the techniques are suitable for all ages and all physical abilities. Most of the techniques will help you to achieve smooth, flowing movement and are beneficial for the free passage of *chi* around the body. Remember never to force your body into any movement—go as far into each step and arm position as you comfortably can. Even if your movements seem slight, with full focus you will still gain the benefits of the exercise.

Fist—*Quan*

Touch the top of your thumb against the nails of your index and middle fingers. Keep the fist hollow and the hand relaxed, as though protecting an egg held in the palm of your hand. The fist position comes originally from martial arts and would once have been clenched. In *Tai Chi* the fist must be hollow to allow *chi* energy to circulate.

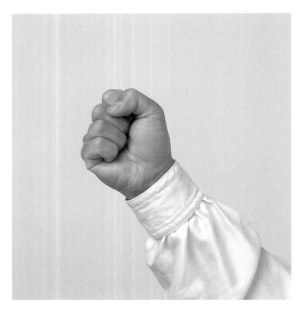

Above:
WRONG: Here, the fist is held in the wrong, clenched position.

Right:
CORRECT: Here, the fist is held in the correct, open position.

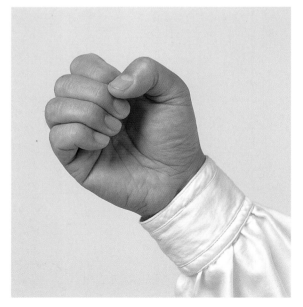

Palm—*Zhang*

When held still, the hand should open naturally, with the first finger, and then the other fingers, spreading slightly so that they are not held tightly together. Allow your little finger to stand forward slightly from the other fingers. Open your thumb and relax it, holding it loosely at an angle away from the palm to create the *hu kuo*, the "tiger's mouth," between the thumb and index finger. Throughout your movements, keep your finger and thumb positions the same, whatever the angle of the wrist.

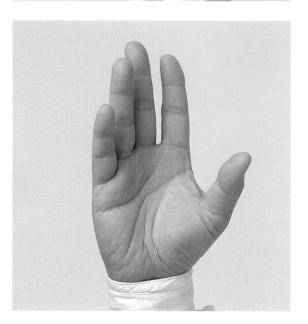

Left:
WRONG: Here, the palm is held in the wrong, stiff position.

Below, left and right:
CORRECT: Two views of the palm held correctly—loose and open.

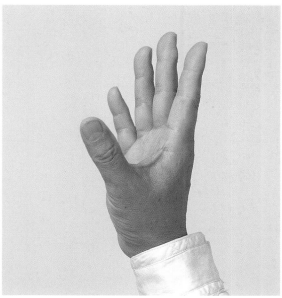

Holding the ball—*Bao qiu*

Because the hands should replicate the shape of the *yin yang* pattern (see page 8), they must always move in a circular motion. In almost every transitional movement between two hand positions, the hands face each other as though holding a ball. You can also use the "hold-ball" position with your hands above your shoulders when freezing a moment of movement. Any size ball can be held, right up to a full span of your arms.

Right:
The basic position shows one hand above the other, palms facing each other.

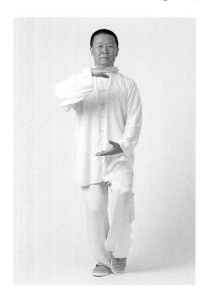
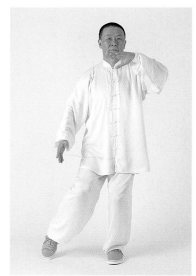

Left:
Normally, you create the "hold-ball" position when turning the body and transferring to the next movement.

Right:
You can also use "hold ball" when both hands are held together, parallel, as you move positions.

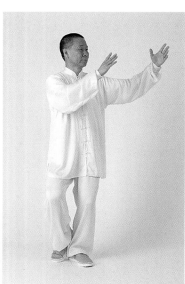
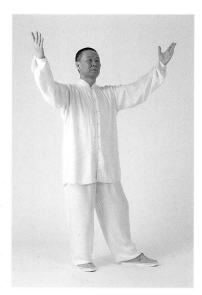

Left:
In addition, you can use the position to hold a huge ball above your head.

Hook—*Gou shou*

First hold out your arm and relax your wrist, letting all of your fingers hang naturally downward. Mimicking the movement of picking something up, close your fingers together. Usually, hold your arm horizontally as you form this hand position, although sometimes you can turn the hook and push your whole arm backwards.

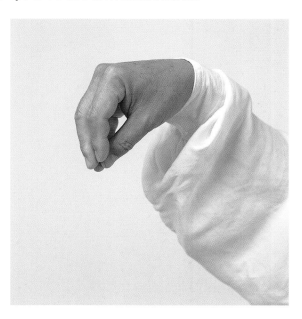

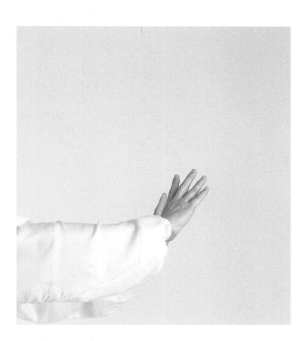

Pushing the hands—*Tui shou*

Hold your hands out in front of you, thumbs pointing toward each other, and imagine you are holding a basketball. Never position your hands with the palms flat forward. The energy for the push should come through your whole body—imagine you are pushing a mountain—not just from your arms and hands. Keep your body upright, never lean forward, with your elbows slightly bent to keep a perfect roundness in your arms. This allows the *chi* to circulate.

Concentrate on your *dan tian—Yi shou dan tian*

The *dan tian* is the center of the body, positioned two inches (five centimetres) beneath and behind the belly button. Throughout *Tai Chi* practice you should concentrate on this spot. All movements start from here—the legs and arms only follow. Never think "leg forward," instead think "*dan tian* forward."

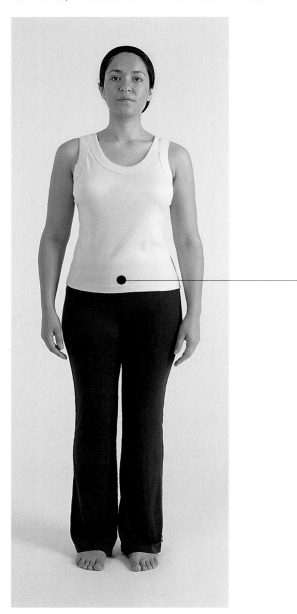

dan tian

Bow stance—*Gong bu*

Keep your spine straight, head and body upright, shoulders relaxed, hips down. Bend the front leg until the knee is directly above the toes, and the back leg until it is straight. Keep your rear heel off the same line as the front one. The front foot should point forward, while the rear heel stretches backward, forcing the body to face directly forward. Check that the heels are not on the same line and your feet are not at too great an angle to each other.

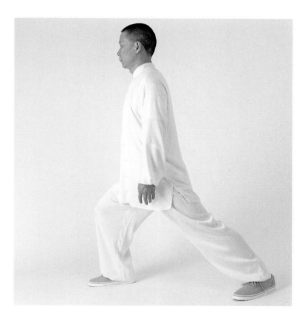

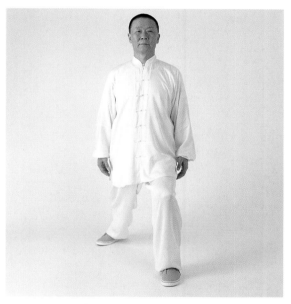

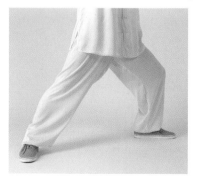

Above:
Position the front knee directly above the toes and keep your back leg straight.

Above:
Stretch the back heel to ensure the body faces fully forward.

Left:
WRONG: If your right heel does not stretch back, the toe will point out to the side—and your body will follow.

Riding-horse stance—*Ma bu*

During *Tai Chi* it is important to center yourself. Keep both feet slightly wider than shoulder-width apart, toes facing forward. Bend your knees forward until they are in line with your toes. Keep your hips flexible, with your torso and head upright, shoulders relaxed. Look straight ahead.

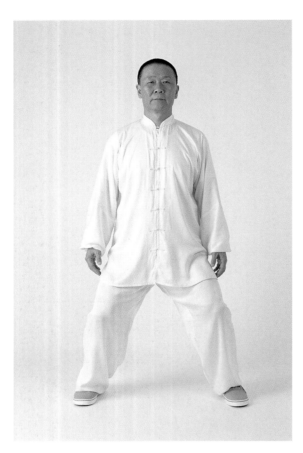

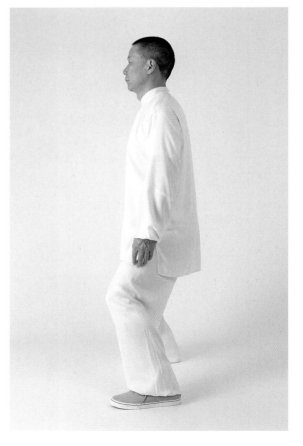

Above:
Stand loosely with your hands by your hips and your feet spread slightly wider apart than the width of your shoulders.

Right:
Check that your knees are over your toes and your bottom is over your heels.

Empty step—*Xu bu*

Use this step when the body's weight is supported completely by one leg, with the big toe of the other leg just touching the ground. Keep the raised leg completely free and flexible so that it is able to go either forward or back at will. Both your torso and your head should be straight.

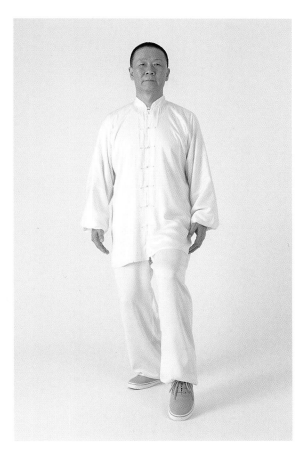

Above:
All your weight should be on your back foot—don't even use the front foot for balance.

Right:
Bend your back leg so that it can absorb the shifts in weight caused by the hanging leg and keep your balance.

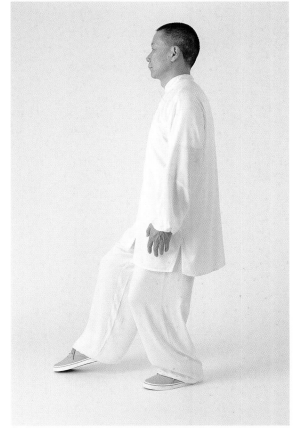

T step—*Ding bu*

To transfer weight from one foot to the other during a Form, take a half-step forward (see below). Sometimes, the T step can lead into the empty step (see page 33).

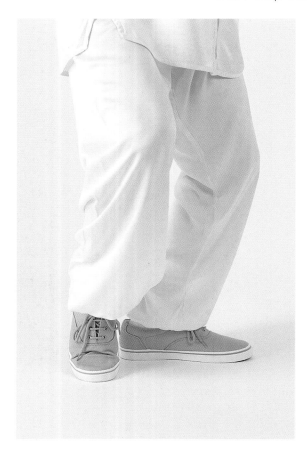

1 Take a half-step forward to bring your feet together. Keep them at right angles to each other and find your balance using the toe that is touching the ground.

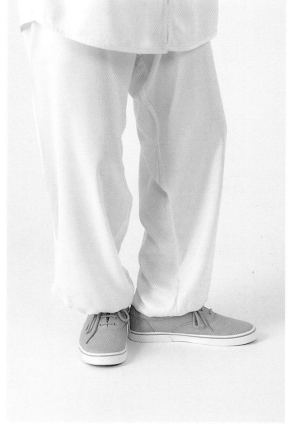

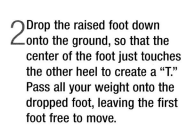

2 Drop the raised foot down onto the ground, so that the center of the foot just touches the other heel to create a "T." Pass all your weight onto the dropped foot, leaving the first foot free to move.

Down step—*Pu bu*

This is a lower stance, with almost seventy per cent of the body's weight held by the bent leg. As this movement was developed as a defence from a high attack, the head should turn to the direction of the outstretched leg as the body drops. When dropping into this position, never force your leg or groin to stretch too far.

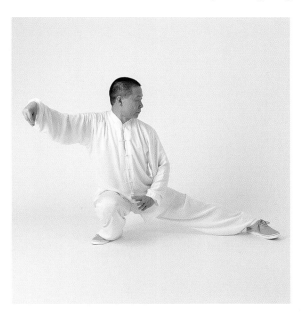

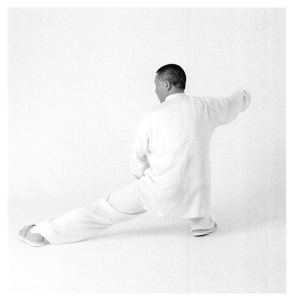

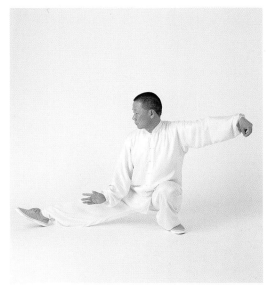

Above:
Hold one hand out in a hook (see page 29) and position the other in front of you at knee height.

Right:
Look back along your shoulder, keeping your body facing sidewise. Your feet should be slightly splayed.

Above:
Only drop as far as is comfortable for you—never overstretch or pull your muscles. If you exercise regularly your muscles will gradually loosen.

Warm Up

Whenever you practice *Tai Chi* you should always start by warming up the body in order to loosen the muscles. Most often practitioners begin their *Tai Chi* exercises after periods of inactivity—first thing in the morning, just after waking, or after many hours at work. It is important to restore flexibility in the body before undertaking any form of exercise in order to prevent strain or injury.

The 12 sections of the Warm Up enable every joint and muscle to be stretched and moved. They ready the circulation for the more strenuous exercise of the *Tai Chi* Forms so that blood can pump quickly to working muscles. By improving the body's flexibility, you can avert most injury problems. Remember: never force or overstretch your muscles—work gently and gradually, and never push to your muscles' maximum extent.

Leg stretch

At the beginning of the exercise session, it is important first to stretch both legs. This allows the ligaments and muscles of the back, pelvis, and legs to warm up and ease into activity.

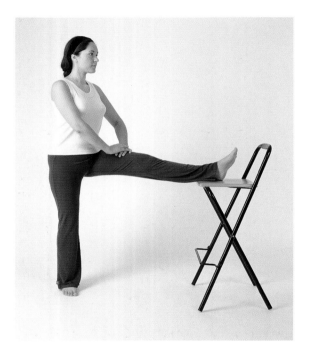 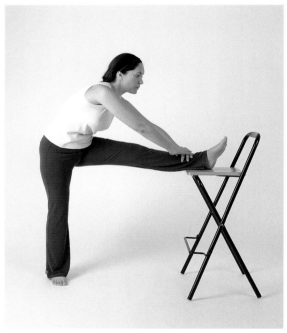

1 Find somewhere 24–36in. (60–100cm) high (such as the seat of a chair) on which to rest your foot. Begin with your left leg, straightening it and placing both hands on the top of your thigh.

2 Keeping the leg straight, slowly bend your body forward. Stretch to your maximum potential, count to eight twice. Change leg and repeat the whole exercise.

Hands and wrists

Next loosen the hands and wrists, and aid your circulation. Start by standing in a comfortable, relaxed position with your feet shoulder-width apart and your hands hanging loosely by your sides, elbows slightly bent.

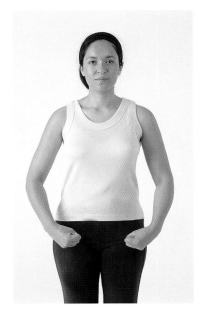

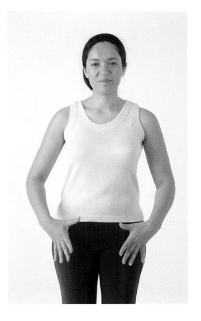

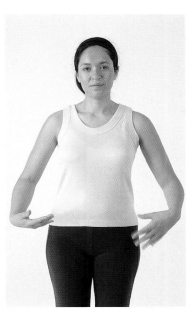

1 Clench both hands into fists, and count to two.

2 Open your hands wide, and count on to four. Repeat the whole clenching and releasing movement four times.

3 Relax both hands and shake them vigorously.

BEGINNING WARM UP: HINTS AND TIPS

• *Tai Chi* is similar to many Western activities, particularly dance. Like them, a major cause of injury can be a failure to warm up adequately before each session.

• When you start exercising, never force any part of yourself. As you practice, your muscles will lengthen over time.

Neck 1

The neck is the vital link at the top of the spinal column, but it is also relatively weak. It is more important to prevent injury here than almost anywhere else in the body. Begin loosening the muscles with the simplest of exercises.

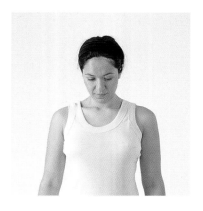

1 Lower your head forward as far as it will go.

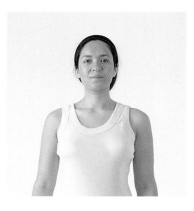

2 Bring it back to its normal upright position, and count "One, two."

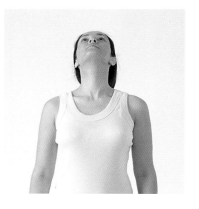

3 Push your head as far back as possible, counting "three," then return to center, counting "four."

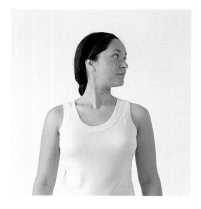

4 While counting "five, six," turn your head as far to the left as is comfortable and then return to center.

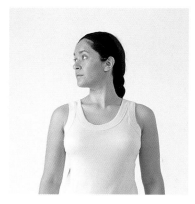

5 Turn to the right and return, counting "seven, eight." Repeat the entire exercise once more.

Neck 2

Once loosened, the neck is ready for more strenuous activity. The continual, circular motion of this warm-up exercise will help to strengthen the muscles and tendons running up the sides of the neck.

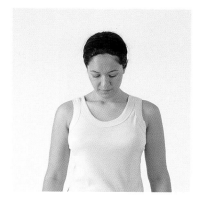

1 Lower your head forward as far as is comfortable.

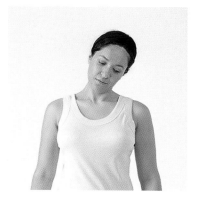

2 Turn your neck in a circle. Start on the left side, move down, to the right, and up.

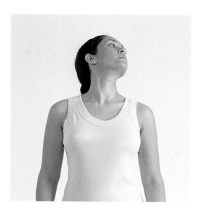

3 As you move, count from one to four and focus on stretching your neck muscles. At "four" you should be looking straight ahead again.

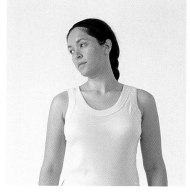

4 Repeat the movement, this time moving first to the right and counting from five to eight. Finally, repeat the entire exercise.

Shoulders

Loosen the shoulders, collar bones, and upper arms by circling your shoulders. This seemingly gentle exercise also prepares many of the muscles of your upper back. Always follow this warm up with the one opposite.

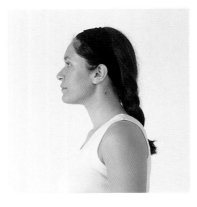

1 Stand straight with your arms hanging loosely by your sides.

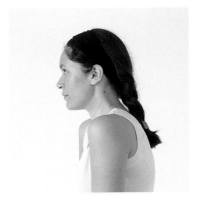

2 Keep your torso and head still. Push your shoulders up and forward in a circular motion.

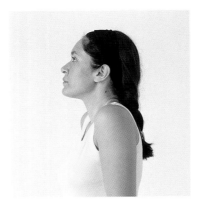

3 Continuing down, back and up, create a full circle. Count from one to four during the whole movement (steps 2 and 3).

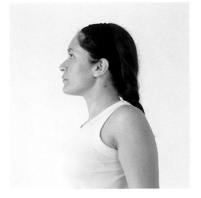

4 For the count of five to eight, make the circle in the opposite direction: Shoulders pushed up and back, then down, to the front and up. Repeat the entire exercise.

Shoulders and back

Synchronize your shoulders with your upper back by stretching them forward and up. Continue the warm up by stretching and turning to the sides to incorporate the muscles of the lower back.

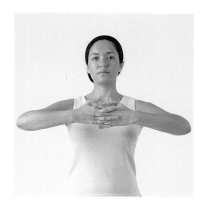

1 Interlock both hands at chest height, palms facing inward.

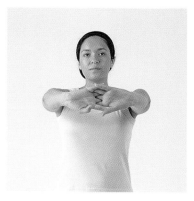

2 Turn your palms out. Push forward; breathe in. Turn them back; exhale. Count "One, two."

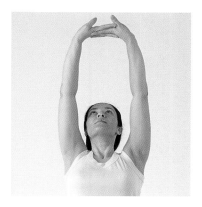

3 Push upward, palms out. Breathe in; return. Breathe out and count "three, four."

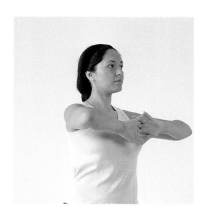

4 Keeping your feet still, turn to the left with your hands against your chest.

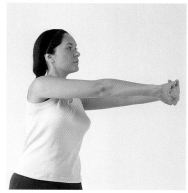

5 Push out, breathing in. Return, breathing out. Count "five, six."

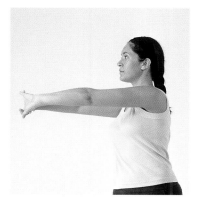

6 Repeat, this time turning to the right. Count "seven, eight." Repeat the whole exercise.

Waist

Now combine your loosened lower back with your waist in a more extensive warm up that will stretch your sides. This warm up will release any trapped tension from the *dan tian* (see page 30)—the area that leads all *Tai Chi* movement.

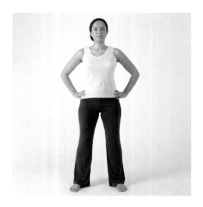

1 Stand with both hands holding your waist. Relax your legs and hips, feet slightly apart.

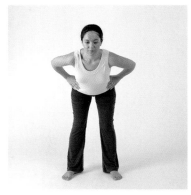

2 Slowly bend the body forward at the waist as far as is comfortable.

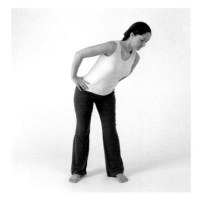

3 Turn to your left, keeping your hands on your hips.

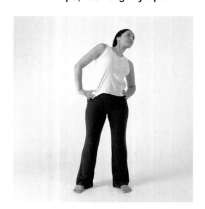

4 In a circular movement, follow round to the left and backward, stretching the length of your back.

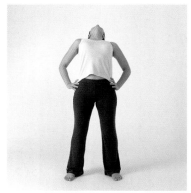

5 Lean as far back as possible, being careful never to overstretch.

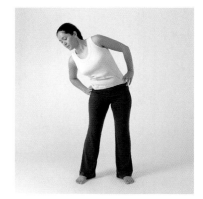

6 Continue through to the right side. Return to the starting position. Repeat three times; then in reverse four times.

Knees

Knees 1: Many of the steps and leg positions used during *Tai Chi* Forms involve more strength than you might imagine. As a result, it is very important to ensure that the knee joints are supple, and the muscles of the calf and thigh are warm.

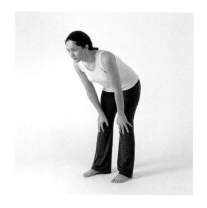

1 Place your feet shoulder-width apart and bend forward naturally, resting your hands on your knees.

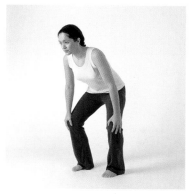

2 Open your knees out and forward, counting "One, two."

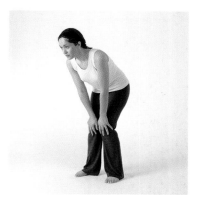

3 Counting "three, four," close the knees inward and push them forward. Return to your original position.

Knees 2: The second knee exercise stretches the hips and ankles, as well as warming up the knees.

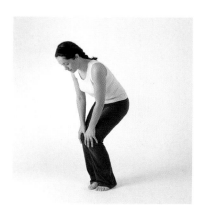

1 With your feet together, hands on knees, move your knees in a counterclockwise circle, counting "One, two."

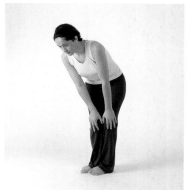

2 Reverse, making a clockwise circle, counting "three, four." Repeat both steps.

Legs

When the parts of the leg have been warmed up during the knee stretches, you can stretch your whole leg and spine a little further. You should now be able to bend more deeply, but still take care not to overexert any joint or muscle.

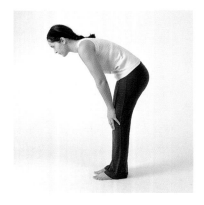

1 With your feet together and your legs straight, place your hands on your knees and bend your body forward.

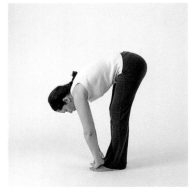

2 Bend until your hands touch your toes, or as near as is comfortable, and hold, counting "One, two."

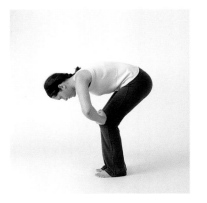

3 Bring your hands back onto knees and bend your knees slightly.

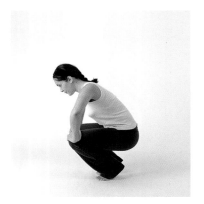

4 Squat down, lifting your heels off the floor, counting "three, four."

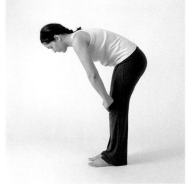

5 Stand up again until your legs are straight. Repeat the exercise once more.

Ankles

The final joint of the leg to be warmed up is the ankle. Take care not to place too much pressure on the toes as you turn the foot—the toes should do no more than act as a pivot. Wear shoes to protect them if necessary.

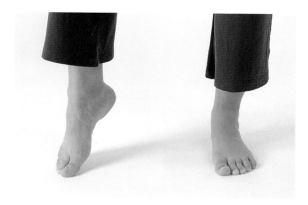 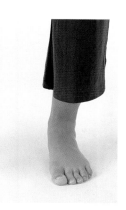

1 Standing on your left foot, raise the right foot until only the big toe is touching the floor.

2 Keep your big toe on the floor. Turn your foot in a circle, counterclockwise, from the ankle. Repeat four times.

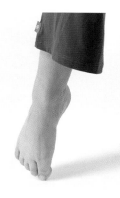 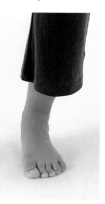

3 Now turn the foot clockwise four times. Repeat steps 1 to 3 once more. Then repeat the whole warm up, standing on the right foot.

Hips—straight

When stretching your hips, keep your torso and neck straight, and your head facing forward. Drop into a bow stance (see page 31), always keeping your spine in line with your back leg.

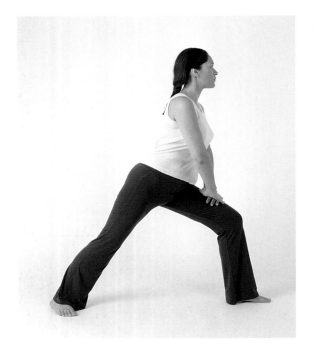

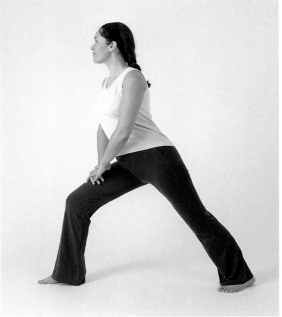

1 Stand in the bow stance position (see page 31) with the left leg forward. Place both hands on the front knee, and lower your body down as far as you can comfortably go. Count from one to eight and release.

2 Turn your body to reverse the position, with your right leg now leading. Place your hands on your right knee. Lower as far as you can go. Count to eight. Repeat the whole exercise once more.

Hips—side

Only stretch as far as is comfortable during this exercise. There is no particular distance to reach—benefit is gained merely from stretching toward your own personal limit. Never over extend yourself—in time your muscles will loosen.

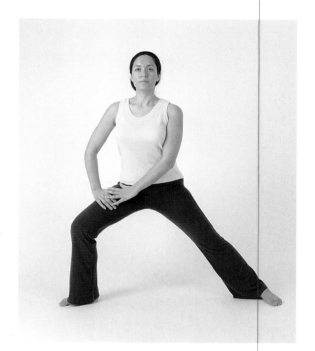

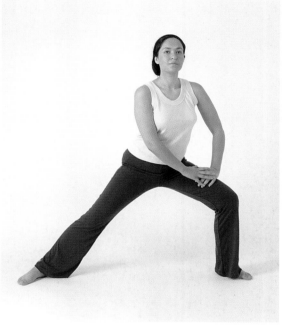

1 Drop into a down step (see page 35)—left leg straight, squatting on the right leg. Stretch downward and count to eight.

2 Change leg and repeat. Repeat the whole exercise once more.

PREPARING TO PRACTICE: HINTS AND TIPS

• Originally a martial art, *Tai Chi* requires every part of the body to be flexible, and capable of fighting, so be sure to start your practice only when you have warmed up thoroughly.

• As your warm up moves to a close, pay particular attention to the hip movements (above): the quality and smoothness of many of the Forms depends on the suppleness of the hip joints.

The 24 Forms

The 24 *Yang*-style Forms that are described here are the ideal introduction to both the philosophy and the physical benefits of *Tai Chi*. The Forms were developed in the 1950s to be a basic but complete combination of the many strands of *Tai Chi*. All the movements of the many strands of *Tai Chi* have been incorporated—and are an ideal basis for extending the study of the art. By studying each Form you will also learn to relax, to control your body, and your mind. Break each one down into its individual movements. Practice each part of the exercise until your body has achieved balance before creating a single flowing stream that recreates the Form.

Form 1
"COMMENCING FORM"

This Form benefits your whole body, acting as a gentle introduction and an ideal preparation to the 23 Forms that follow. Remember throughout to hold your chest and neck straight. Keep the *chi* held well down in the *dan tian* (the center of your body; see pages 19 and 30) by breathing deeply, naturally, and smoothly.

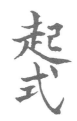

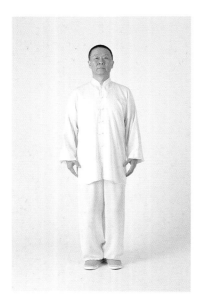

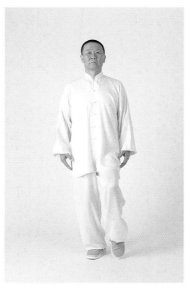

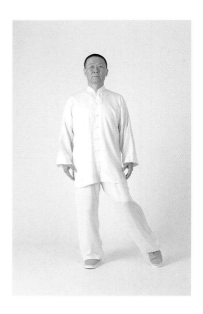

1 Stand upright with your heels together, toes open naturally, spine straight, shoulders relaxed, and arms hanging loosely. Look straight ahead with relaxed eyes.

2 Inhaling, let your body weight drop down naturally by slightly bending your knees before lifting up the left heel, moving all your weight onto your right side.

3 Move your left foot out so that it is shoulder-width distance from the right foot.

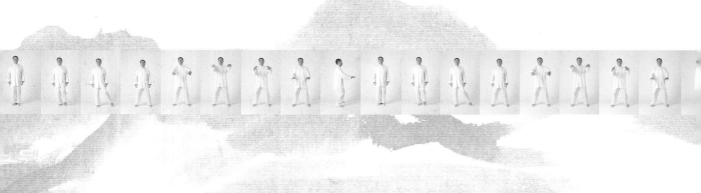

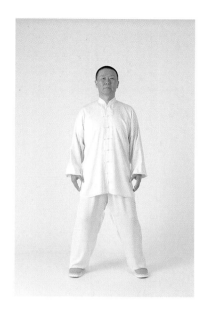

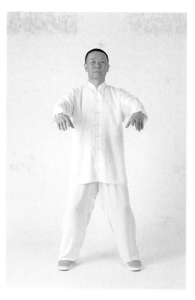

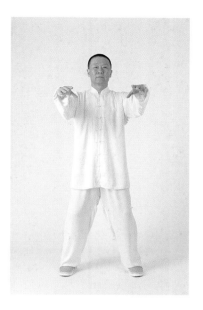

4 Exhaling, move your body to the center, while concentrating the mind.

5 Breathing in, raise your arms slowly keeping the palms of your hands facing downward.

6 Keep raising your arms until they reach shoulder height.

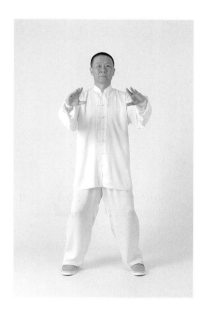

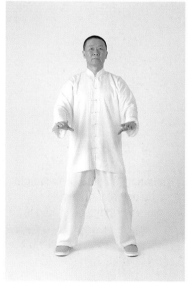

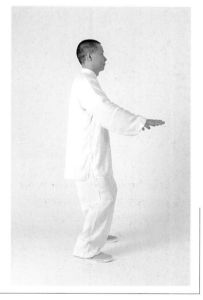

7 Breathing out, bend your knees while pressing your palms downward.

8 Let your elbows drop until your hands press down at the level of your *dan tian* (see side view, right).

Always keep your torso erect and spine straight. Keep your chin in, even when you are bending. When the tension is in your knees, keep your waist and hips relaxed and your shoulders and elbows down.

Form 2

"WILD HORSE PARTS MANE THREE TIMES ON BOTH SIDES"

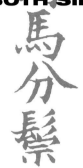

When the hands separate, the energy from the *dan tian* (see page 30) can start to spread to every part of the body. Stretching in the bow stance (see page 31) in steps 13 and 17 opens the meridians (the passageways through which *chi* flows) to the ends of the limbs and through the muscles.

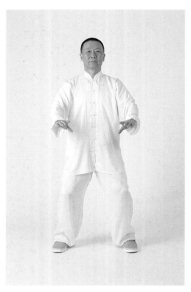

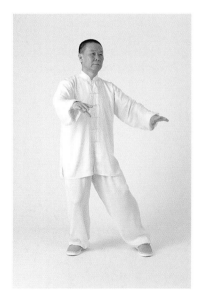

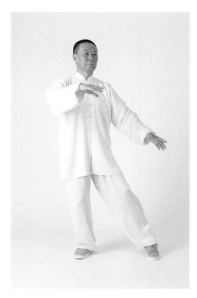

1 Start by standing in a relaxed position with your feet shoulder-width apart. Let your arms and hands fall to the front. They should not be completely relaxed—hold them as though you are pressing down a piece of board underwater.

2 Inhale, keeping your knees slightly bent. Begin to raise your right hand in front of the right side of your chest, while turning at the waist to allow the right leg to straighten.

3 Take all the weight off your left foot. Raise your left heel as your right arm comes up to the horizontal and your left hand moves out in a downward curve.

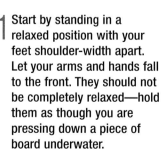

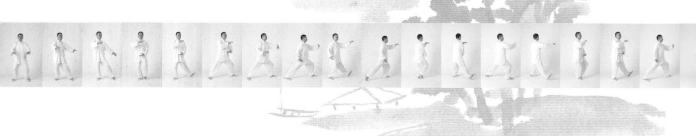

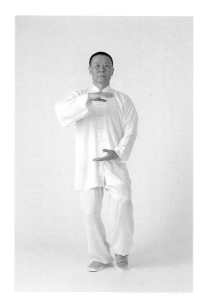

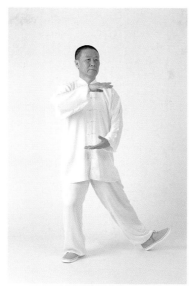

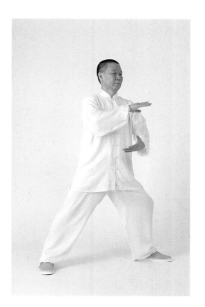

4 Move to your right, turning back to face the front. Place the left foot beside the right, knee bent, toes touching the floor. Hold the hands in the "hold-ball" position (see page 28).

5 Keeping the weight on the right leg, place the left foot out, heel to the floor first. Keep the body facing forward with the arms moving in opposite directions.

6 Breathe out while gradually transferring your weight onto your left foot while both arms move across your body. Bend your left knee.

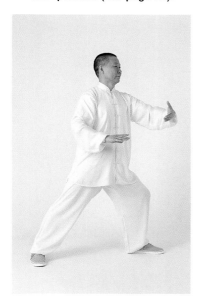

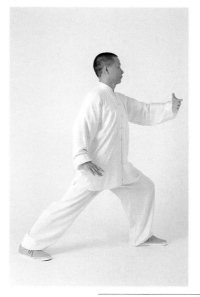

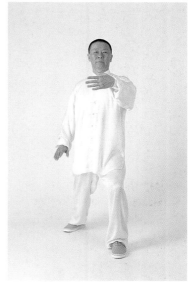

7 Turn your body to the left at the waist to align with your outstretched foot. Keep your weight over your bent, left knee.

8 Turn your body, raising your left hand to in front of your chest, palm inward (see alternate view, right). Lower your right hand to beside your hip. Keep your left knee bent to end the first stage.

Viewing the same position from straight ahead shows that you keep your feet in a straight line, holding your left hand in front of your chest and directly above your knee.

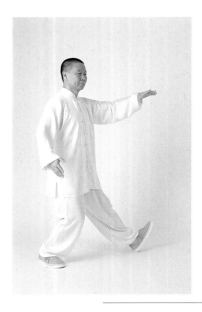

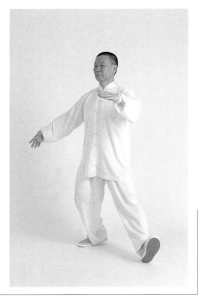

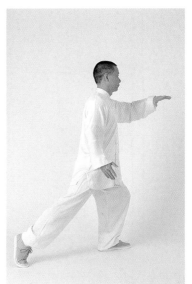

9 Inhaling, sit back slowly, shifting your weight onto your right leg (see alternative view, right). Raise the toes of your left foot and turn them outward.

As you transfer your weight, keep your body upright, moving from below the waist and using your right hand for balance.

10 Bend your left leg and turn your body left and forward, shifting the weight onto the left leg. The right hand naturally follows the body movement.

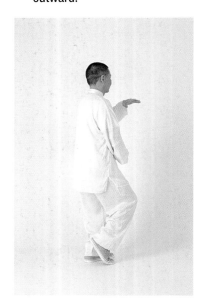

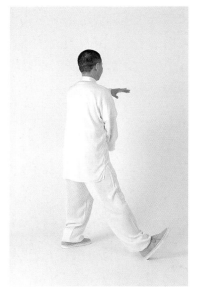

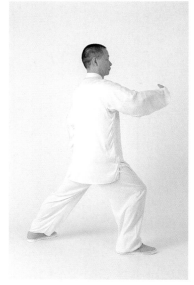

11 Standing on the left leg, allow the right toes to touch the ground with the arms in the "hold-ball" position, left hand on top.

12 Breathing out, move the right foot a step forward placing the heel on the ground first.

13 Transfer your weight forward into the bow stance (see page 31) with the palm of your right hand facing in, elbow slightly bent. Press the left hand down, palm downward.

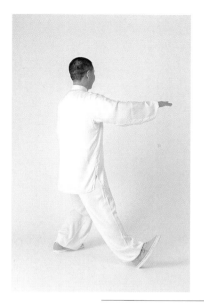

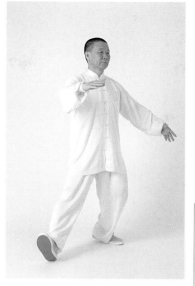

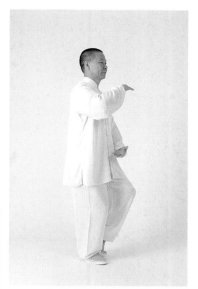

14 Inhaling, sit back slowly, shifting your weight onto your left leg (see alternative view, right). Raise your right toes and turn them outward.

As you begin the final stage of the Form, remember to follow the previous movements in reverse. Begin by swinging your left hand in towards your waist.

15 Move your body weight forward into the "hold-ball" position again, taking all the weight on the right foot.

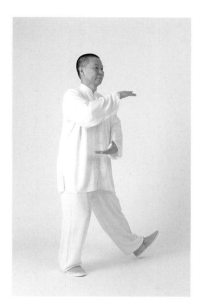

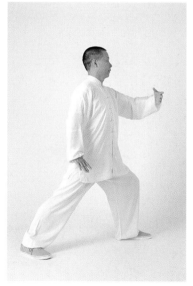

HINTS & TIPS

• When your body drops into the bow stance, first turn the waist to lead the shoulder and hand as they stretch out.

• When the hands are in the "hold-ball" position, keep the top elbow pointing down.

16 Once again place your weight on the back, right leg with your left foot out.

17 Finish in the bow-stance position with your weight forward, and turning at the waist. It is important to stretch the rear heel to make sure the body is facing properly forward.

Form 3

"WHITE CRANE FLASHES ITS WINGS"

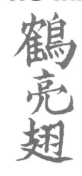

Move your weight downward while the *chi* travels upward. Finish with both arms held in a sinuous, curved "S"-shape that contrasts with the straightness of your back.

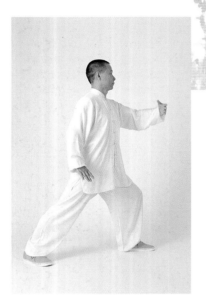

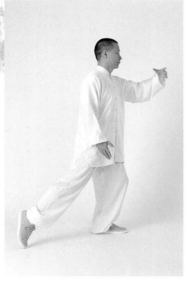

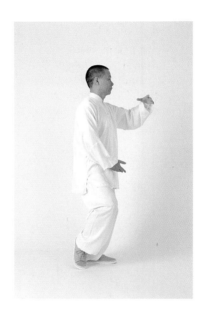

1 Begin in the bow-stance position (see page 31) which ended the previous Form.

2 Inhaling, lift the back heel and begin to turn the right hand to face the left.

3 Continuing to turn the arms, move the body half a step forward, placing the toes of the right foot by the left heel.

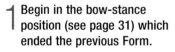

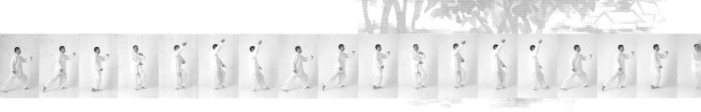

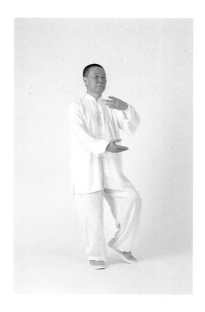

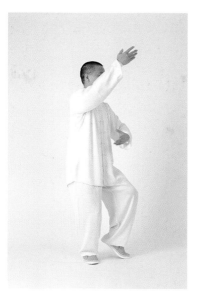

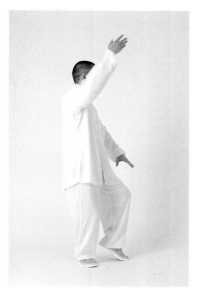

4 Ground the right foot, transferring your weight to it, and lift your left heel, all the time turning the body slowly round to the right.

5 Look straight ahead while you raise your right hand, palm in, and drop your left. Keep your feet in the same position as step 4.

6 Exhaling, turn your body to the front while your arms continue moving, all the time keeping the weight on your right leg and your left foot forward.

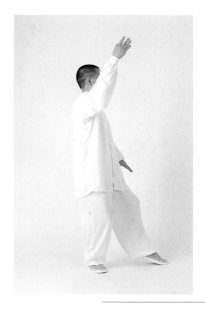

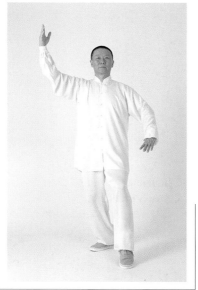

7 Raise the right hand, palm inward, past your temple while the left hand moves in front of your hip, palm downward (see alternative view, right).

The front view shows that both elbows should be bent at similar angles with your hands held away from your body.

Form 4

"BRUSH KNEE ON BOTH SIDES THREE TIMES"

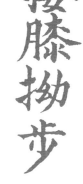

One of the most important factors to remember in *Tai Chi*, and especially this Form, is to allow every movement of the body and arms to be led by the waist. Never let your arms pull your body around: let your body swing your arms.

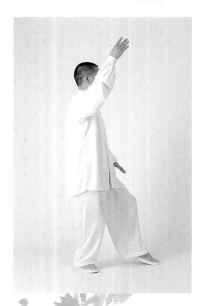

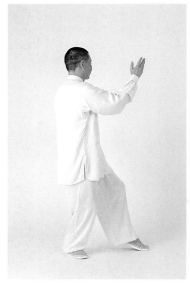

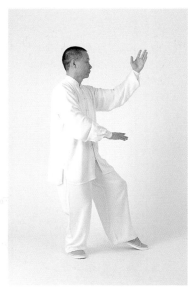

1 Begin in the position that ended the previous Form—right arm raised and weight on your right leg. The toes of your left foot are placed gently on the ground in an empty step (see page 33).

2 Taking a big breath, turn your torso slightly to the left, your right hand moving down while your left hand moves up.

3 Turn back to the right, with your right hand circling past your abdomen. Your left hand moves in a curve up and to the right, across your face.

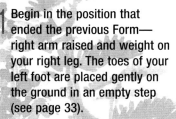

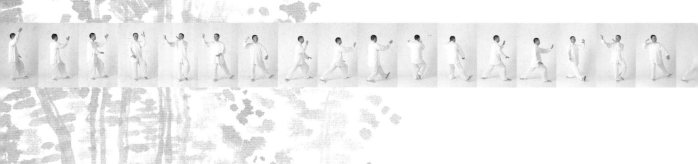

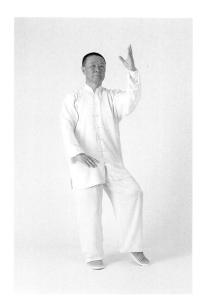

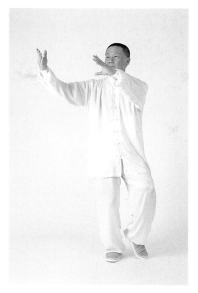

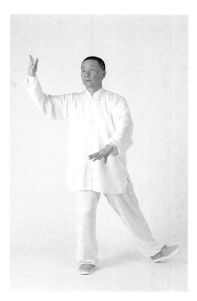

4 Your waist now acts as an axle, leading your arm in a curved movement, as the body turns to the right.

5 Continue to raise the right hand to ear height, keeping your arm slightly bent; the left hand crosses the chest. As the two hands face each other, look at your right hand.

6 Move your left foot outward as your left hand continues to move across the front of your body and presses down.

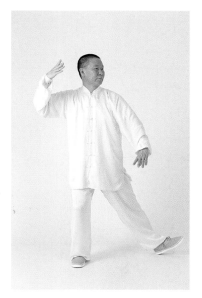

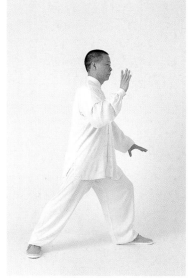

7 With your left heel touching the ground, your right hand moves leftward by the side of the ear and your left hand falls downward.

8 Using your waist turn your body left, with your left hand by your knee. Watch the path of your right hand and transfer your weight forward into the bow stance (see page 31). Push your right hand forward.

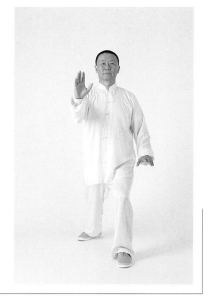

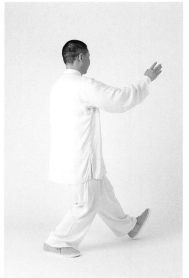

9 When your right hand is fully extended, stretch your right heel to ensure that your body is facing straight ahead, ending the first movement (see alternative view, right).

From this angle, you can see that the left hand should face downward and be close to your hip. Your right hand faces forward.

10 Inhaling, sit back slowly, bending your right knee and shifting your weight onto your right leg. Raise the toes of your left foot and turn them slightly out.

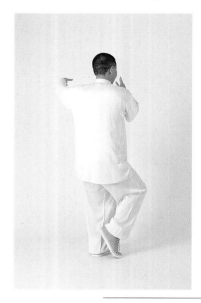

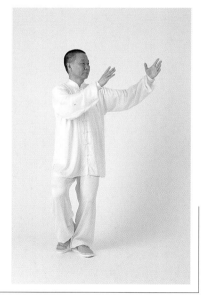

11 Shift your weight to your left leg by moving your body forward and slightly left, and bending your left leg. As your two hands face each other, look at the left hand (see right).

As your left heel gently touches the ground, your right hand draws leftward by the side of the ear and the left hand falls downward.

12 Step out with the right foot. As your right heel touches the ground, your left hand draws rightward by the side of your ear and your right hand falls down to the side of your abdomen.

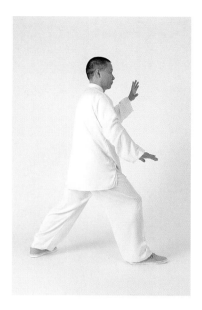

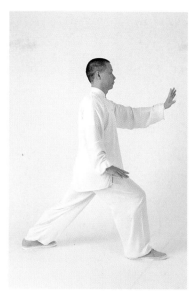

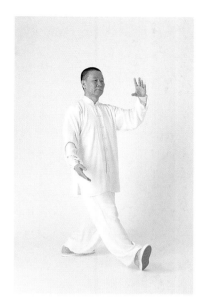

13 Turn right at your waist while your weight moves forward, with your right hand above your right knee and your left hand starting to push forward.

14 Transfer your weight forward, coming into the bow-stance position, pushing your left hand forward and your right hand down.

15 Inhaling, sit back slowly, bending your left knee and shifting your weight onto your left leg. Raise the toes of your right foot and turn them slightly outward.

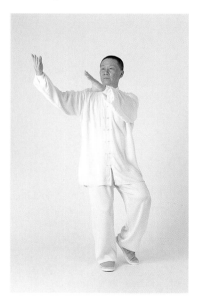

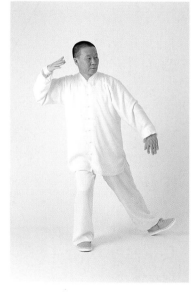

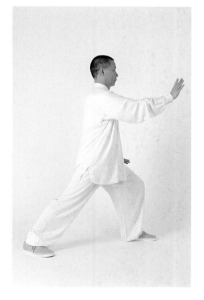

16 Move your body forward and slightly to the right, bending your right leg and shifting your weight across. As your two hands face each other, look at your right hand.

17 Exhaling, step out with the left foot. As the left heel touches the ground, the right hand draws past the ear while the left hand falls down toward your left knee.

18 Turn your waist leftward while transferring your weight forward into the bow-stance position. Push your right hand forward and your left hand around your knee to your side.

Form 5

"STRUM THE LUTE"

揮琵琶

Whether your body is moving forward or backward, your torso should always be held upright, with a straight spine. Most importantly, when your limbs are stretched out to the front and back, an upright body allows you to move fluidly into the next position and keeps your *chi* held down in your *dan tian* (see page 30).

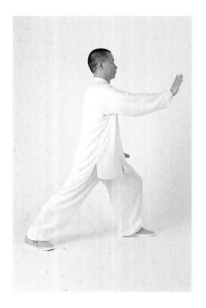
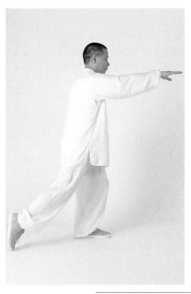
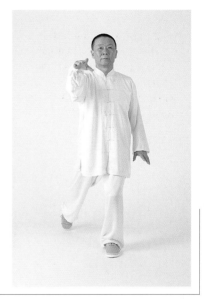

1 Begin in the position that ended the previous Form, in the bow-stance position (see page 31), with your right hand extended forward and your left hand by your side.

2 Breathing in, move your weight onto your left leg, extending your right arm, with your hand flat (palm down), pressing down with the left hand (see alternative view, right).

From this angle you can see that you should stretch the fingers of your right hand forward while the left hand remains still.

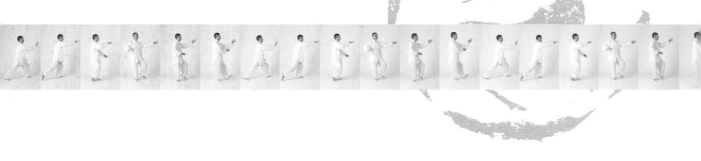

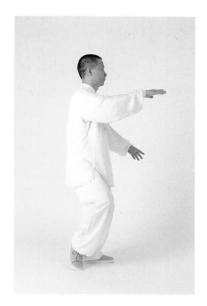

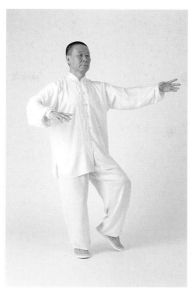

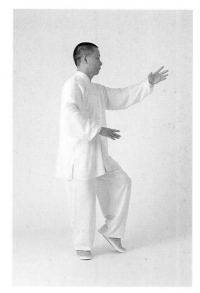

3 Half-step your right leg forward to stand in a T step (see page 34), starting to bring your right arm back toward your body. Swing your left arm up and forward.

4 Shift the weight onto your right leg and lift your left heel. At the same time, turn your waist to the right to pull your right arm backward and bring your left arm forward.

5 Exhaling, start to turn back to the left, squeezing both the left elbow and right hand inward and forward.

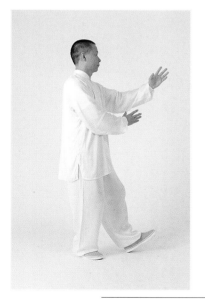

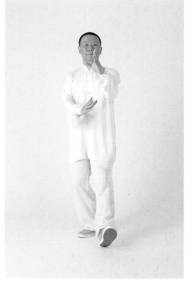

HINTS & TIPS

• Whether moving forward or back, your torso should remain upright: never lean forward.

• Your arms move forward or back only in response to movement from the waist.

6 Lifting your toe and turning your left foot out slightly, finish with your left heel touching the ground and your arms held in front of you in the "strum-the-lute" position (see alternative view, right).

Finish with your left hand in front of your face and your right hand directly beneath it.

Form 6

"CURVE BACK ARMS ON BOTH SIDES FOUR TIMES"

When stepping backward never stand with your feet in line with one another to give you good balance. Also, keep your the body held at the same height as you move backward and forward through the different movements of the Form.

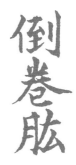

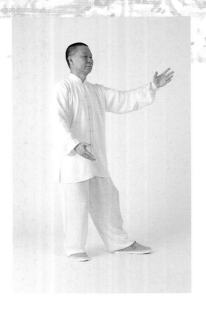

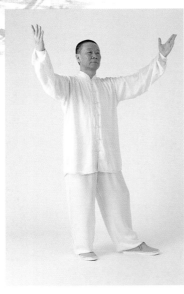

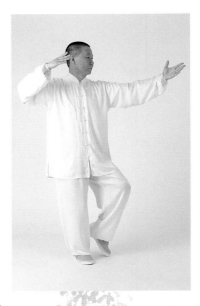

1 Beginning in the position that ended the previous Form, start to swing your body to the right and drop your right hand.

2 Inhaling, hold both hands, palms up, above eye level with your arms slightly bent.

3 Shifting your weight to your right side, lift your left heel, and bring your right hand up by your ear.

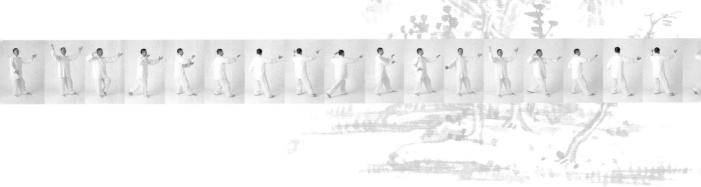

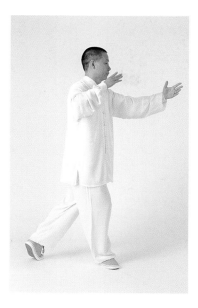

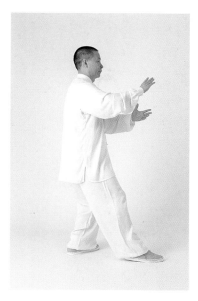

4 Breathing out, take a step backward with your left foot, continuing to turn your body to the left, all the while watching your left hand.

5 Lean back and push out your right hand, palm downward, while drawing your left hand back, palm up.

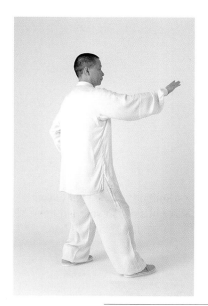

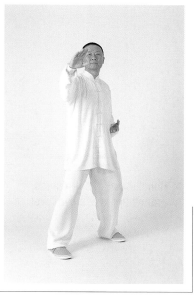

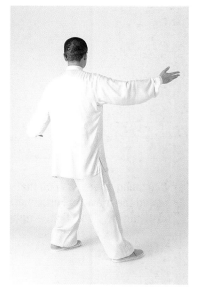

6 Watch your right hand stretch forward as your left hand reaches waist level. Ensure your feet are parallel and your left arm is held close to your body to end the first movement (see alternative view, right).

From this angle, you can see that both feet are parallel, and the right hand is directly over the right foot.

7 Turn your body to the left, dropping your left arm, and turning over your right hand so that your palm faces upward.

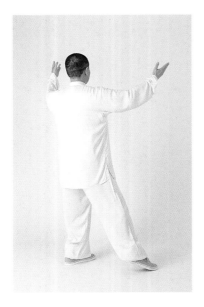

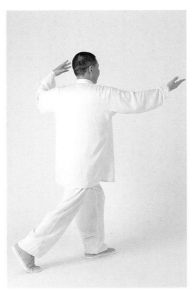

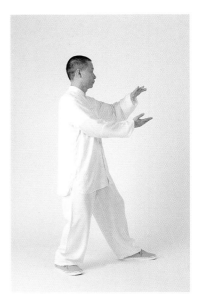

8 Inhaling, open your stance by lifting your right heel, as your left hand swings up to shoulder level, palm up. Turn your right hand so that it is also palm up.

9 Take a step back with your right foot, turning your body to the right, repeating your earlier movement in reverse— now watching your right hand.

10 Lean back and push out your left hand, palm downward, while bringing your right hand back, palm up.

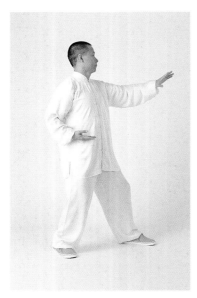

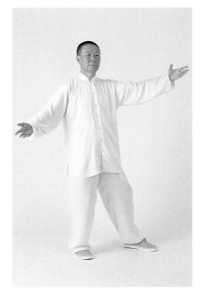

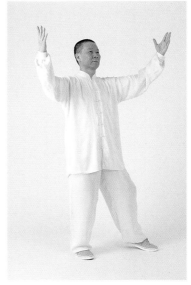

11 Watch your left hand as it extends and your right hand reaches waist level, ending the second movement of the Form.

12 Open your stance, turning your left hand over, and opening out your right hand.

13 Inhaling, lift both hands, palms up, to eye level.

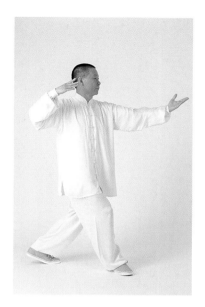

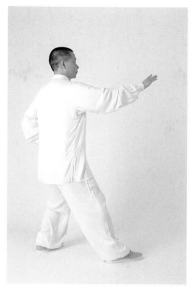

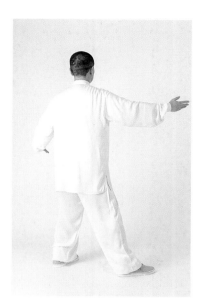

14 Exhaling, take a step back with your left foot, turning your body to the left, repeating your earlier movement on the other side, watching your left hand.

15 Lean back and push out your right hand, palm downward, while raising your left arm with the hand palm upward, ending the third movement.

16 Turn to the left and open your left arm outward.

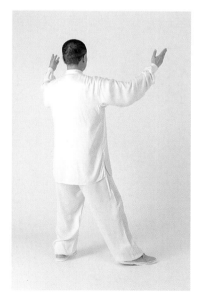

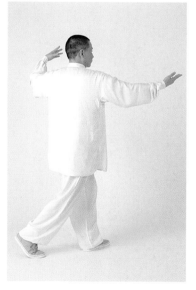

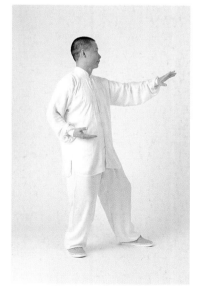

17 Inhaling, open your stance, lifting both of your hands up to eye level.

18 Breathing out, take a step back with your right foot, turning your body to the right, repeating your earlier movement on the other side—this time watching your right hand.

19 Extend your left hand and keep your gaze through it as your right hand drops to waist level, ending the Form's fourth movement.

Form 7

"GRASP THE BIRD'S TAIL, LEFT STYLE"

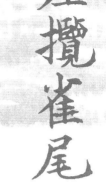

左攬雀尾

In this Form especially keep in mind that, whether the body is turning to the left or the right, or travelling backward or forward, all movements should be led from the waist. At all times remain slow and smooth, and let your movement aid your balance. In *Tai Chi*, you should never be jerky or forced.

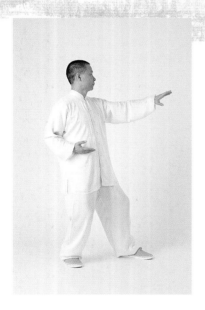

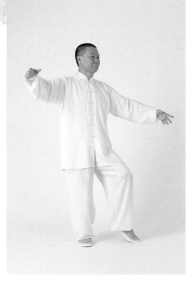

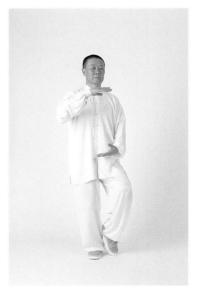

1 Begin in the position in which you ended the previous Form.

2 Inhaling, swing your body slightly to the right, bringing your left arm up to shoulder level and your right arm across the lower part of your chest. Slowly shift your weight onto your right leg. Raise your left heel.

3 Move into the "hold-ball" position (see page 28) and place your left toes by your right foot.

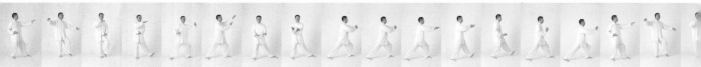

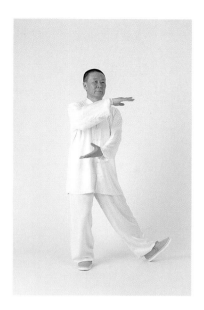

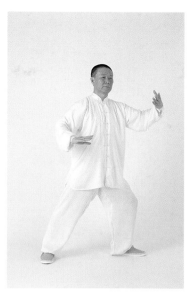

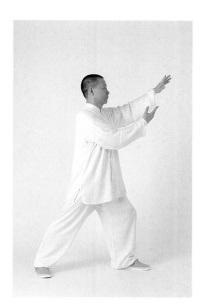

4 As you move through the "hold-ball" stance take a step across to your left.

5 Exhaling, move into a bow stance (see page 31). Bring your left arm across your chest and drop your right arm in a circular movement across the right side of your chest.

6 Turn to the left at the waist to send both arms forward, your left hand as if parrying a blow while turning the palm out. As your right arm reaches chin height, turn your palm inward.

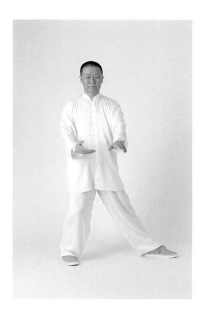

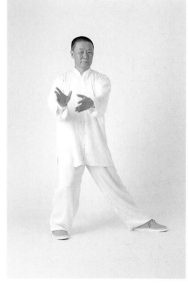

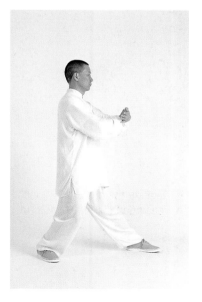

7 Shift your weight backward and turn to the right, while moving both hands downward in a stroking motion.

8 Circle both hands across your stomach by turning them over and twisting both wrists. Rest the fingers of your right hand on your left wrist.

9 Breathing in, twist to the left as both hands cross.

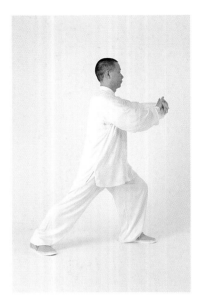

10 Breathing out, shift your weight forward and push both hands away from you.

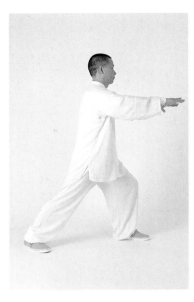

11 Separate your hands and turn them so that your palms face downward.

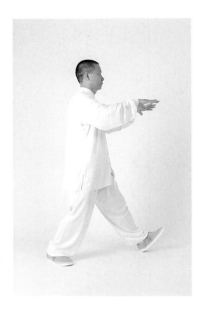

12 Inhaling, lean back onto your right foot, using your left heel for balance, and bring your arms back in toward your body.

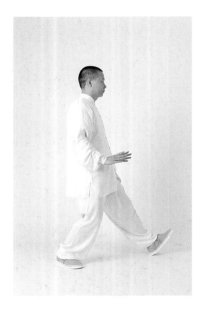

13 As you reach the extent of your backward lean, press your hands down in front of your stomach.

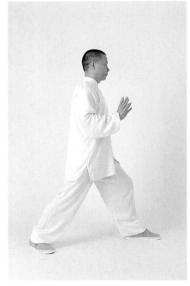

14 Breathing out, immediately shift your weight forward slightly, bending the left knee and putting your left foot flat on the floor, and raise both hands to chest height.

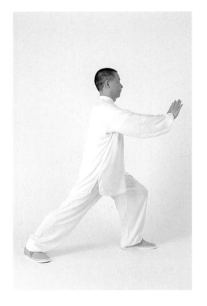

15 Shift your weight forward into a bow stance (see page 31), while pushing your hands forward.

Form 8

"GRASP THE BIRD'S TAIL, RIGHT STYLE"

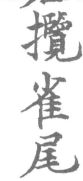

Ensure that your hands and feet coordinate both with each other and with the rest of your body. Good balance is determined by the timing of your arms and legs and the positioning of your toes as you move from one stance to the next.

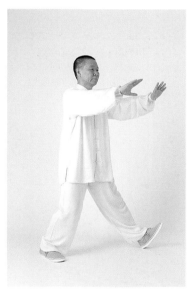

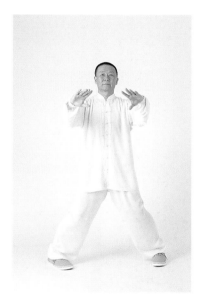

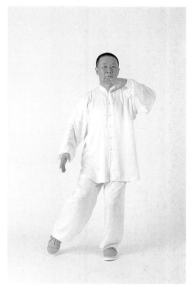

1 Commencing from the position in which you ended the previous Form, lean back onto your right leg, lift the toes of your left foot and start turning to the right.

2 Inhaling, move into the riding-horse stance (see page 32) with both hands remaining outstretched at shoulder height, palms down.

3 Move your body weight onto your left leg while swinging your right arm down and turning your hand over (palm upward), pulling your left hand across your throat.

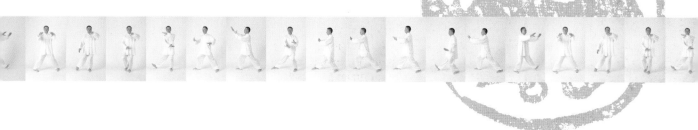

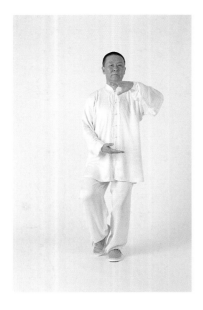

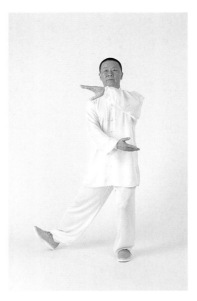

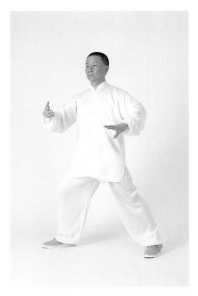

4 Bringing your right foot against your left, move into a "hold-ball" position (see page 28).

5 Stretch your right foot out, heel to the floor, as the "hold-ball" position is broken.

6 Breathing out, lean across to the right while opening both arms.

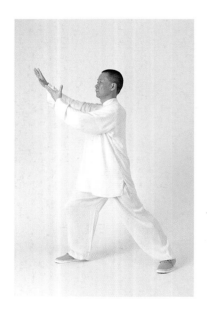

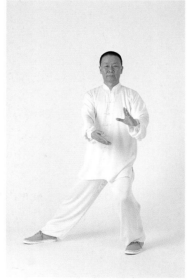

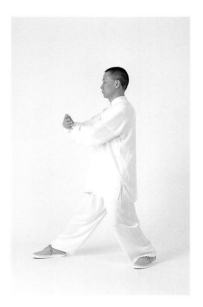

7 Move into a right-footed bow stance (see page 31), while turning the waist to send both arms forward, reaching out to your right—now with your left palm up and right palm down.

8 Inhale, leaning across to your left, and turn your body to face the front. While your hands stroke down across your chest, twist both wrists.

9 Cross your left fingers over your right wrist and turn back to the right, lowering the toes of your right foot as you do so.

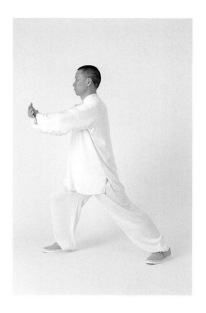

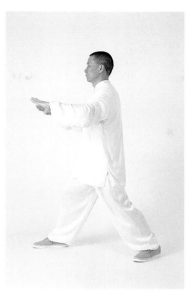

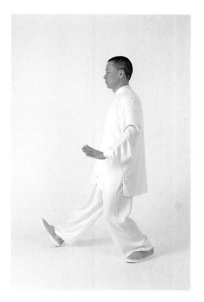

10 Exhaling, move into a right-footed bow stance, pushing your hands out at shoulder level.

11 Open your hands, palms downward, and begin to move your weight backward.

12 Place your weight on your left foot, using your right heel for balance and bring your arms back into your body at waist level.

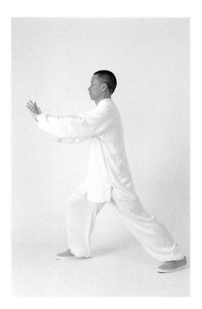

13 Exhaling, raise your hands to chest height while shifting forward again into a right-footed bow stance. Push your hands forward at shoulder height with your palms forward.

HINTS & TIPS

• Keep your torso straight, using your waist as a pivot.

• Keep the movements of your body, hands, and feet evenly paced.

• Step out to the side softly—like a cat.

• Always look in the direction of the movement and let your hands follow naturally.

• Your breathing should match your movements: never hold it or let it become rushed.

Form 9

"SINGLE WHIP"

Keep your torso upright, with your shoulders relaxed, and elbows down. Use your hooked hand (see page 29) to balance your body, especially when leaning into the bow stance (see page 31) at the end of the Form—the steadier you hold it, the smoother the Form.

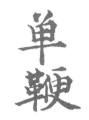

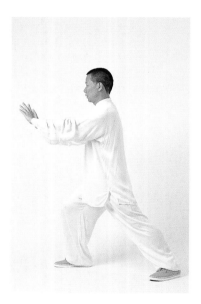

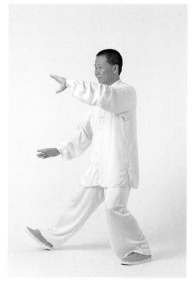

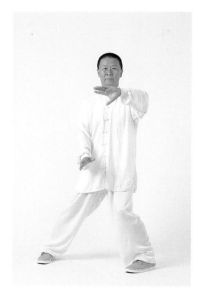

1 Begin in the position in which you ended the previous Form— a bow stance (see page 31) with the right knee bent and both hands pressed outward.

2 Breathing in deeply, move your body weight to the left, lifting the toes of your right foot and turning them inward, while also turning the right hand.

3 Continue turning your body to the front, dropping your right hand down as the left hand swings naturally across your chest.

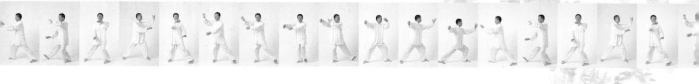

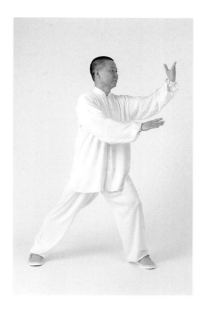

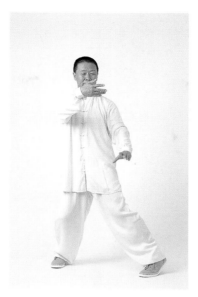

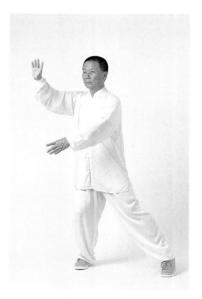

4 Keep your feet in position as your body turns to the left, both arms following to the left.

5 Without moving your feet, turn your body to the right and stretch both hands back to the left, all the time watching the left hand.

6 Transfer your weight onto the right leg and move the right arm across, as the left arm crosses the stomach. The heel of the left foot is raised.

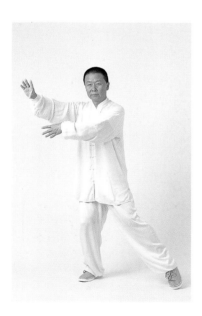

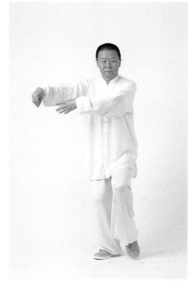

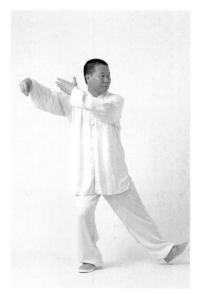

7 Continuing to transfer your weight gradually onto the right leg and bring the left hand up.

8 As you transfer weight onto the right leg, bring your left foot in and, with your right arm at shoulder level, form the hook (see page 29) with your right hand.

9 Move the left foot away from the right foot, toes raised and heel off the floor. Move your left arm up above the front of the right shoulder, palm facing inward.

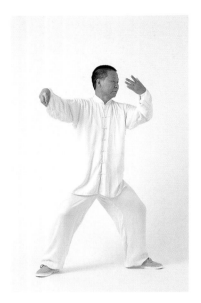

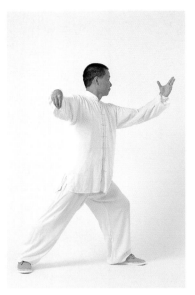

10 Exhaling, turn your body to the left while shifting your weight forward, your left arm naturally following the body's movement.

11 Carry on turning left at the waist, your weight still moving forward, pushing forward and opening the left hand.

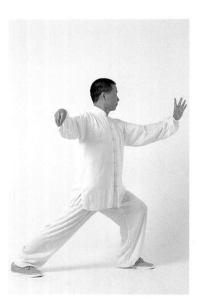

12 Finish the movement in a left-footed bow stance, stretching back your right heel. Ensure your body faces your left with your eyes looking through the fingers of your left hand.

HINTS & TIPS

• Hold in your chest to enable your arms to move in smooth circles.

• Keep both your shoulders and elbows down—don't let them become tense.

• Use your front hand as the line for the direction of your nose. Look through your fingers.

• In the bow stance stretch your right heel back to ensure your body is facing properly forward.

Form 10

"WAVE HANDS LIKE CLOUDS, LEFT STYLE THREE TIMES"

Always use the waist as a pivot when turning the body, with the arms swinging in a continuous, circular movement. Your body should never lean away from the upright. Control your breathing. Repeat the movement on opposite sides.

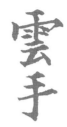

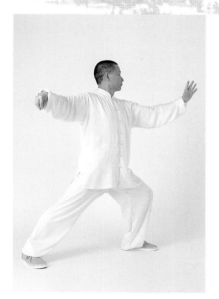

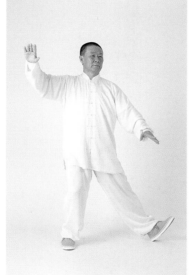

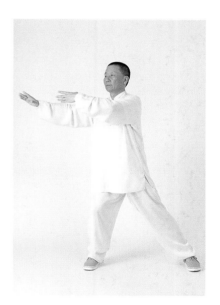

1 Begin in the position in which you ended the previous Form—in a left-footed bow stance (see page 31) with your left arm horizontal and your right hand in a hook (see page 29) as you look through the fingers of the left hand.

2 Breathing in deeply, lean onto your right foot, pivoting on your left heel, while curving your left arm down and across your body, and opening your right hand.

3 Turn your body to the right at the waist, turning your left toe inward, while lifting your left arm in an arc across your body and beginning to drop your right hand. Keep watching your left hand.

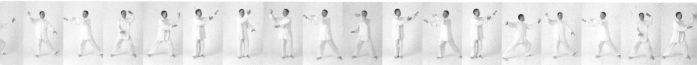

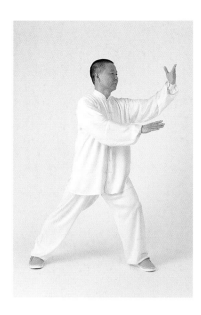

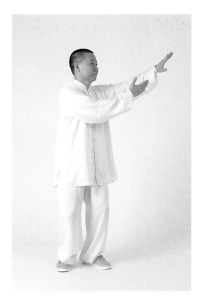

4 Shift your weight back onto both feet as you continue the arc made by your left arm above your shoulder. Your right arm drops toward your waist, palm down.

5 Keep your feet in position as your body turns to the left, both arms following to the left.

6 Breathing out, step to the left as your right arm reaches shoulder height. At the same time, twist both hands (left palm moving down, right palm up), to end the first movement.

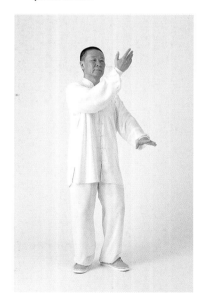

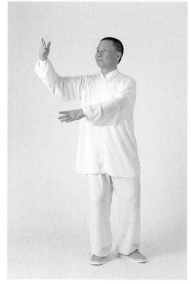

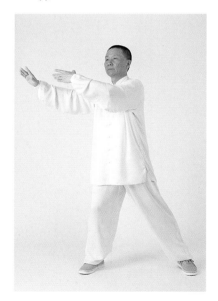

7 Breathing in, shift your gaze, following your right hand as as you continue to bring it up across your face. Drop your left arm. Let your body begin to turn naturally back to the front.

8 Turn again to the right as your right arm arcs away from you and you lift your left hand up in front of your chest.

9 Step across to the left as your hands sweep past each other at shoulder height. Remember to keep turning the palms and now look back to the left hand.

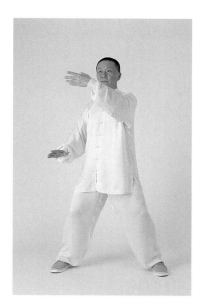

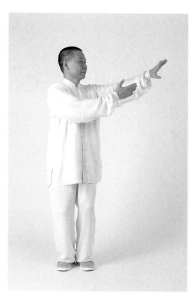

10 Breathing out, turn back to the center, ensuring your weight is evenly distributed in the riding-horse stance (see page 32).

11 Continue repeating the sequence through a turn to the left. Return to the center, ending the second movement.

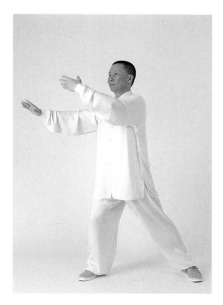

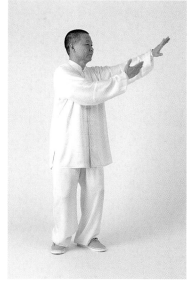

12 Repeat the entire Form to the left once more.

13 End when you are stretched once again to the left with your feet together.

Form 11
"SECOND SINGLE WHIP"

The positions of the arms and legs should mimic each other in this Form—don't press out your left hand any further than you step across in the final left-footed bow stance (see page 31). Follow the movements of the previous Single Whip (Form 9; pages 76–78), ending with a right-handed hook (see page 29).

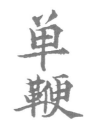

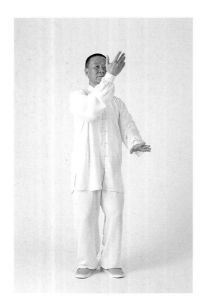

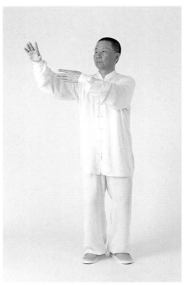

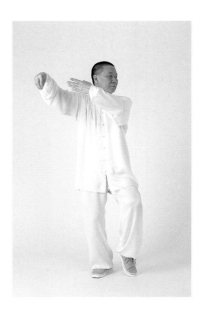

1 Begin in the position in which you ended the previous Form—with your feet together, left hand raised with the palm facing in, and your right hand downward, palm facing the floor. Begin turning to the right.

2 Inhaling, watch your right hand as it passes your face and turns outward. Raise your left hand and turn it inward as it rises over your chest.

3 Making a hook (see page 29) with your right hand, turn your head to the left and lift your left heel, ready to step out.

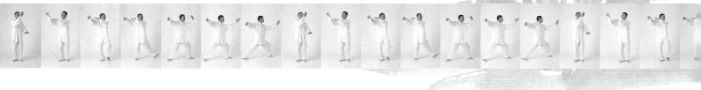

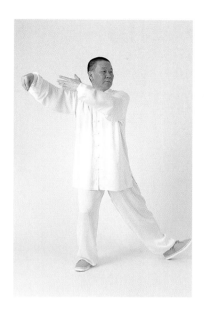

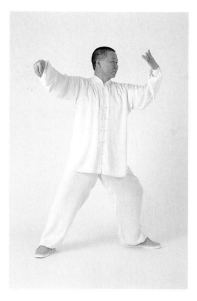

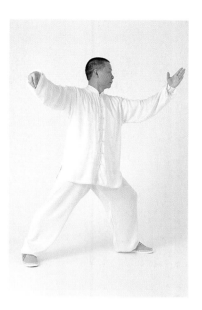

4 Breathing out, step outward with your left foot, placing the heel on the ground first.

5 Moving into a left-footed bow stance (see page 31), keep the hook in your right hand while pushing your left hand forward past your face (palm in).

6 Stretch out leftward, keeping your right hand in a hook and all the time watching your left hand (still with the palm facing inward).

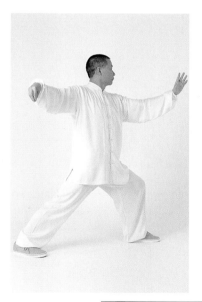

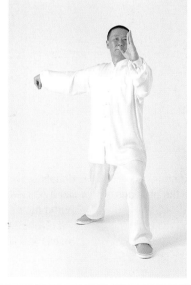

7 Now turn your left hand so that the palm is held open, turned slightly outward, in front of your face (see alternative view, right).

Ensure that your body and left arm are in a straight line. You should be balanced by your hooked right hand.

Form 12

"HIGH PAT ON HORSE"

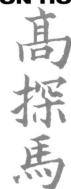

高探馬

Stretch your body, keeping your weight down low around the *dan tian* (see page 30), but allowing the *chi* to rise. Your outstretched arm should always remain slightly bent, don't disrupt your natural balance by stretching too far ahead.

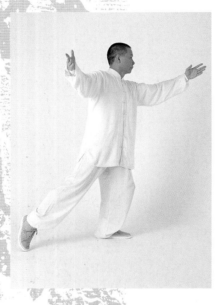

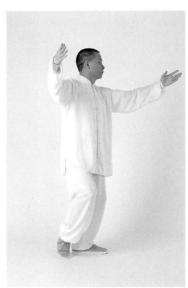

1 Begin in the position in which you ended the previous Form—in a left-footed bow stance (see page 31), with your right hand hooked (see page 29), and watching your outstretched left hand. Start to shift your weight forward onto your left leg.

2 Breathing in, bring your right foot up, resting its toes down beside your left foot, as your hand, palm forward, passes your ear.

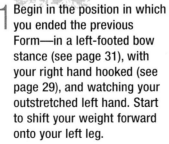

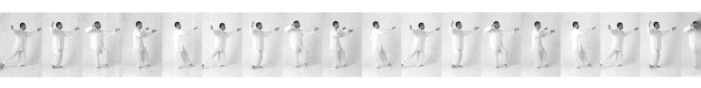

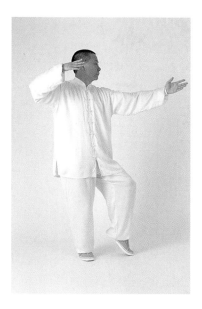
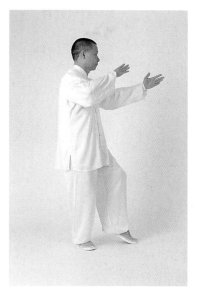

3 Put your right heel on the floor and shift your weight onto your right foot. Lift your left heel and bring your right hand beside your ear, palm down.

4 Breathe out, keeping your left toes on the floor. Pull back your left hand, keeping the palm up. Press your right hand outward at shoulder height, with the palm facing down.

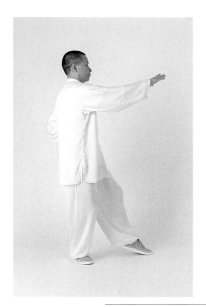
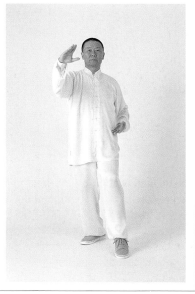

5 Finish in the empty step (see page 33), looking ahead with your right arm extended, keeping a slight bend at the elbow, and your left hand held by your waist, palm up (see alternative view, right).

From this angle you can see that the left elbow is kept in close beside your waist.

HINTS & TIPS

• In the empty step don't put any weight on the left leg—be stable standing on your right leg. Keep both legs bent at all times.

• Stretch your torso throughout, pushing the weight down, but letting the *chi* rise.

• Always keep your right arm curved with the fingers pointing across to the left.

Form 13

"KICK WITH RIGHT HEEL"

In this Form, when the foot kicks out, you must especially concentrate on keeping your body balanced. When preparing to complete the Form, check that your body and neck are perfectly upright and that your left leg stays slightly bent, giving you a firm base. Keeping your eyes focused along the line of your kick will also help steady you.

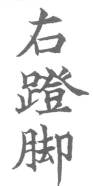

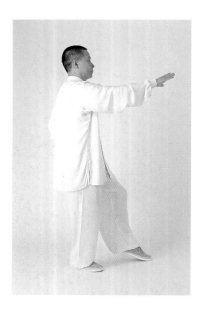

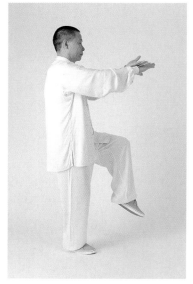

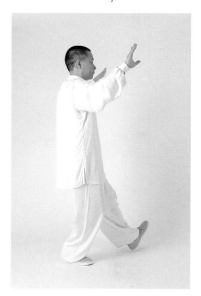

1 Begin in the position in which you ended the previous Form —in a left-footed empty step with your right hand raised, and your left hand by your waist, palm up. Start turning slightly to the right lifting your left hand up and away from your chest.

2 Begin breathing in as you raise your left leg from the floor. Bring your left hand, palm up, across your chest so that it passes over your right hand as you bring your right hand back in toward your chest.

3 Using your left foot, take a step out to the front and side. As the foot touches down, place the heel on the ground first. Circle both hands upward and outward.

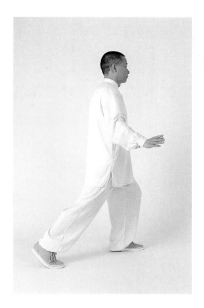

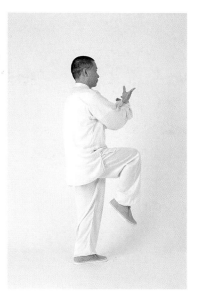

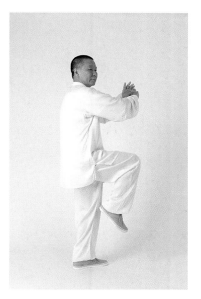

4 Shift your weight onto your left leg, bringing your hands down to waist level. Raise your right foot to bring it alongside your left.

5 Raise your right leg so that your thigh is horizontal. Cross your right wrist over the outside of your left, breathing out sharply.

6 Immediately breathe in again, looking out in the direction in which you will kick. Open out your hands, turning the palms forward as you do so.

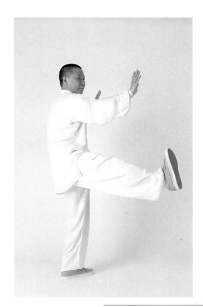

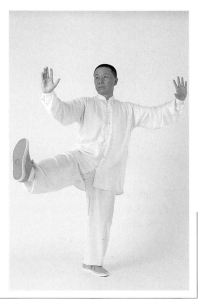

HINTS & TIPS

- Kick out slowly so that you do not lose your balance by making a sudden movement.

- Ensure that both your right hand and your eyes follow the line of your outstretched foot.

7 Finish by exhaling and as you do so fully extend your right leg and stretch out your hands, keeping only a slight bend at each elbow (see alternative view, right).

Seen from the front, the fingers of your right hand should be held open and in line with your raised leg. Look between your fingers.

Form 14

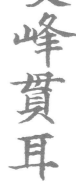

"STRIKE OPPONENT'S EARS WITH BOTH FISTS"

Although *Tai Chi* is now used almost exclusively as a mode of exercise, this Form is a clear reminder that the practice's origins lie in the martial arts. When punching, keep your elbows down and close to your body at all times. The elbows should never swing out. Let the power of the punch come from the shoulders, not the arms.

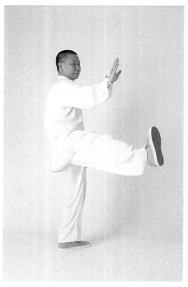

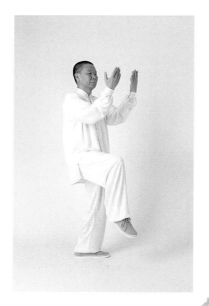

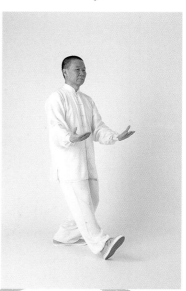

1 Begin in the position in which you ended the previous Form—with your right leg fully extended and your right hand outstretched, looking through the fingers of your right hand. Your raised leg, right hand, and gaze should all be in line.

2 Breathing in deeply, pull back your right foot, keeping the thigh level, and bring both hands up to your face in front of your chest, palms held inward. Turn to the right until you have spun 45° from the previous movement.

3 Exhaling, step forward with your right foot, heel first, and bring both hands down to waist level, palms up.

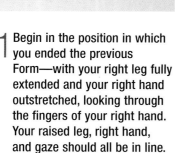

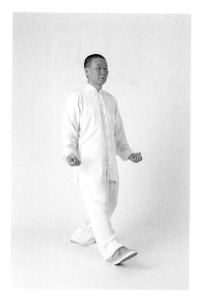

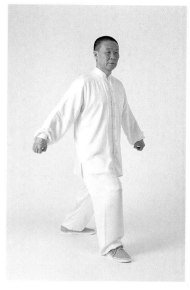

4 Form your hands into hollow fists (see page 26) as you shift your weight slowly forward.

5 Rotate both fists downward, ready to punch in time with your shifting weight as your body moves forward.

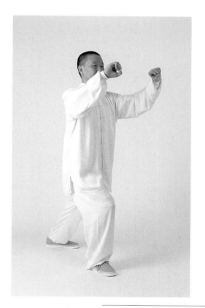

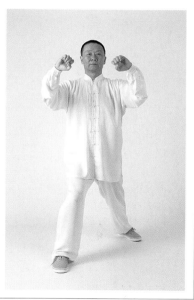

HINTS & TIPS

• The main force of your punch comes from the movement of your body: swing your arms as your body moves forward into the bow stance.

• Your eyes should follow always follow the line in which the toes of your outstretched foot point.

6 Bend your right knee and stretch your left heel, shifting your weight forward to finish in a fully extended bow stance (see page 31). As you do so, bring your fists up to box the enemy's ears on both sides.

In this front view you can see that, when you punch upward, you should keep your elbows well below the level of your hands and held into the body.

Form 15

"TURN AND KICK WITH LEFT HEEL"

When your foot pushes out, imagine that your heel is the contact point of a kick and will the power of the *dan tian* (see page 30) all the way through the leg as it stretches out. Hold the toes upright, at right angles to the leg, to protect them from injury from your imaginary opponent.

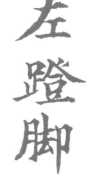

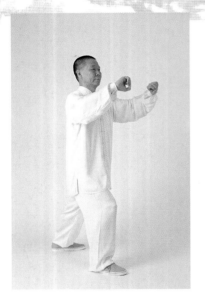

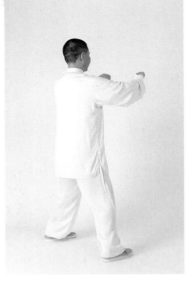

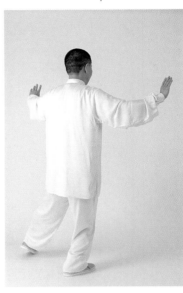

1 Begin in the position in which you ended the previous Form —in a fully extended bow stance (see page 31) with your hands held at eye level in hollow fists.

2 Inhaling, gradually shift your weight onto your left leg and turn your body through 90°, turning the toes of your right foot inward.

3 Shifting your weight slowly across to the right, open your arms out and bring your left foot alongside your right foot.

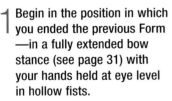

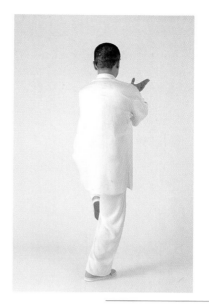 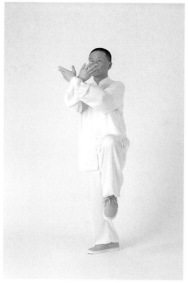 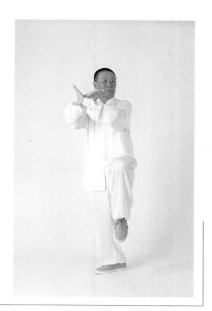

4 Exhaling, bring your hands back across your chest (see right). Lift your left leg, bent at the knee, keeping your thigh horizontal and your toes pointing to the ground.

The front view shows both palms of the crossed hands facing inward, the left hand outermost. Your gaze follows the line of the kicking leg.

Breathing in, turn your head to the left and rotate both hands outward.

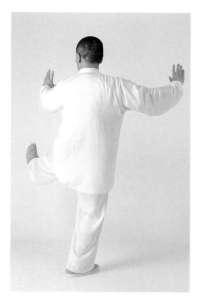

5 Finally, fully extend your left leg and stretch out your hands, keeping only a slight bend at the elbow. This is a chopping stance.

HINTS & TIPS

• Although you are recreating an aggresssive kick, be sure to perform the Form slowly and methodically, lifting and extending your leg with fluidity rather than power.

• Kick out with your heel, and keep your left palm and your gaze in line with your extended leg.

Form 16

"PUSH DOWN AND STAND ON ONE LEG, LEFT STYLE"

When dropping toward the floor, raising your body up, or stepping forward, always avoid leaning away from an upright position. Keep your head up, bottom in, and back straight. Do not worry if you cannot match the depth of the down step (see page 35) shown in this Form: the *Tai Chi* movements should stretch you, but never to extremes.

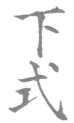

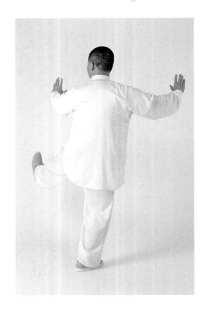

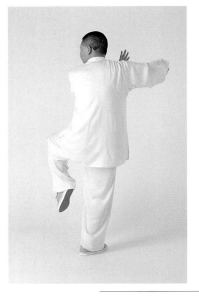

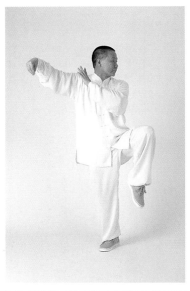

1 Begin in the position in which you ended the previous Form—with your left leg fully extended and your hands outstretched, with a slight bend at the elbow.

2 Inhaling, pull your left foot back, keeping your thigh level and your toes pointing downward. Make a hook (see page 29) with your right hand and bring your left hand across your face (see right).

This front view emphasizes how your lifted toes should be in a vertical line with your shin; and how your hands should be held level to the right side of your head.

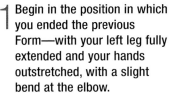

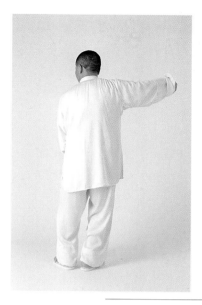
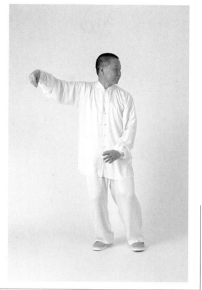

3 Exhaling, step down with your left foot, bringing your feet together. Drop your left hand down in front of your body to your navel (see right).

Your left hand should reach your navel as your left toes touch the ground. The right hand remains in a hook position.

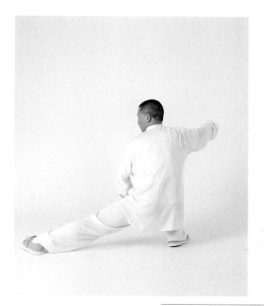
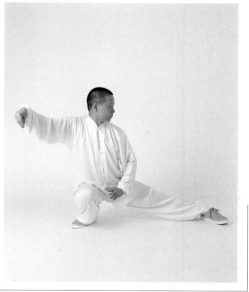

4 Immediately move into a right-footed down step (see page 35) with a straight left leg. Keep your back straight as you drop down. Look to the left. (See alternative view, right.)

In this front view, you can see that the left hand remains in front of the navel and the right hand stays in the hook position throughout the drop into the down step.

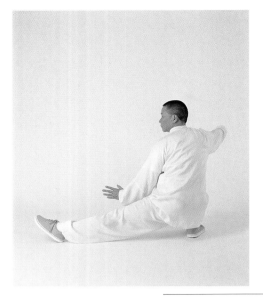

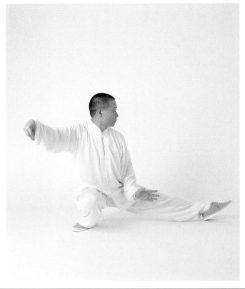

5 Inhaling, turn your left foot out to point forward and rest on its heel. Prepare to stand up. Turn your left hand (see alternative view, right).

Turn your left hand so that it is at right angles to your right leg, pointing toward your left foot.

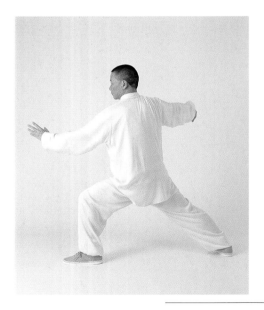

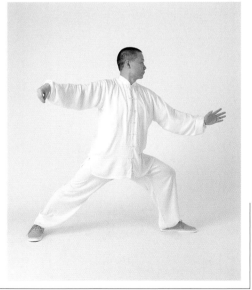

6 Shift your weight forward, bending your left leg and raising your body as you do so. Keep your right hand in a hook (see alternative view, right) while raising your left arm up to chest height.

The front view shows how the right arm remains horizontal with the hand in the hook position and the left toe at right angles to the body—ready to be turned forward before the next movement.

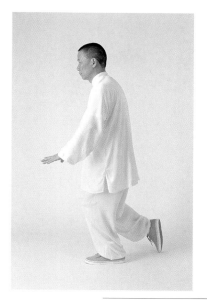
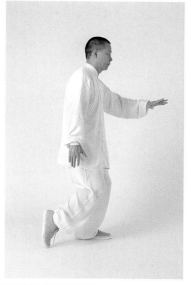

7 Exhaling, turn fully to the right by stepping forward with your right foot, dropping your left hand, palm down, toward your waist and begin sweeping your unhooked right hand forward.

The view from the other side emphasizes how a fluid step up coincides with the dropping of the right arm.

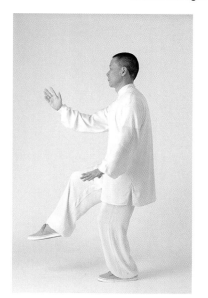
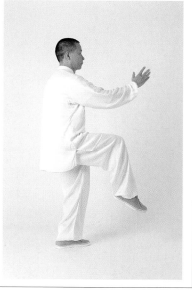

HINTS & TIPS

• When dropping into the down step keep your bottom down and your hips up.

• Keep your elbows down at all times.

• When standing on one leg, ensure that you are fully balanced before attempting to lift your foot off the ground.

8 Raise your right leg while keeping the left leg bent slightly at the knee. Bring your right hand up to shoulder level (see alternative view, right).

The view from this side clearly shows the right hand at shoulder level. Look straight ahead, ignoring your right hand.

Form 17

"PUSH DOWN AND STAND ON ONE LEG, RIGHT STYLE"

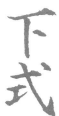

Repeating the previous Form in reverse helps the body to become fully balanced—it is important to ensure that you can create the same level of strength and balance when standing on the right leg as when standing on the left. Look straight ahead, following the direction of the hand as it is held at the beginning of this Form.

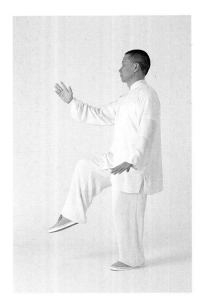
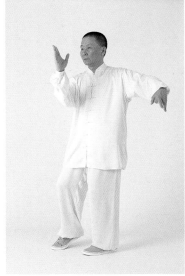
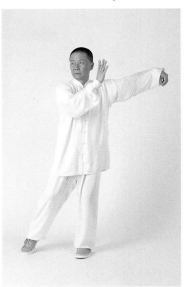

1 Begin in the position in which you ended the previous Form—with your right leg raised, your left leg bent slightly at the knee and your right hand held with an open palm at shoulder level.

2 Inhaling, create the previous form in reverse. Placing your right foot down beside the left for additional support as your body turns to the left, raise your left arm up to shoulder height and backward. Bring your right hand toward and in front of your face.

3 Turn fully round to your left and place your weight on your left leg. Form a hook (see page 29) with your left hand and, as your right hand passes your face, begin to lift your right leg.

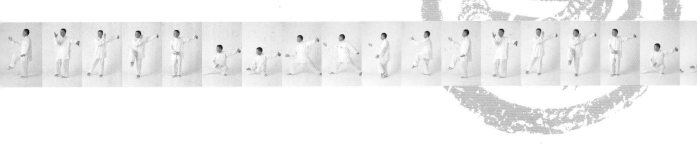

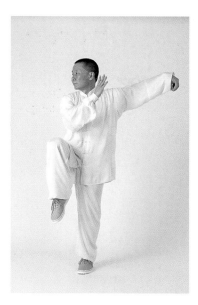

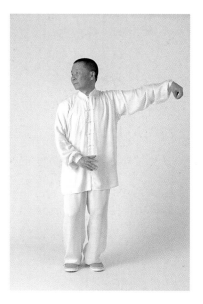

4 Looking to the right, raise your right knee up until your thigh is horizontal, toes pointing down, and start to drop your right hand across your chest.

5 Exhaling, place your feet together as your right hand reaches your navel. Keep your left hand in a hook, steady at shoulder height.

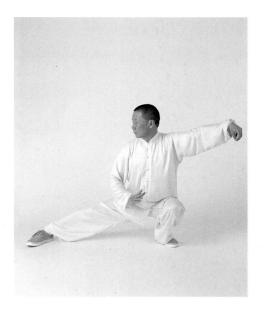

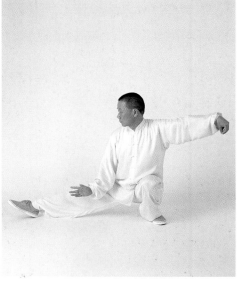

6 Stretch out your right foot sidewise so that your leg is straight and you create a right-footed down step (see page 35). Gaze in the direction of your outstretched foot.

7 Breathing in, turn your right foot outward so that it rests on its heel and turn your right hand in the same direction. Prepare to move forward and stand up.

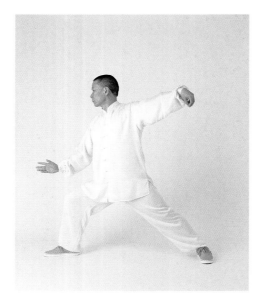

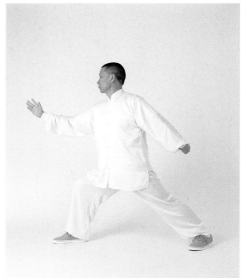

8 Shift your weight forward to raise up into a right-footed bow stance (see page 31). Keep your left hand in a hook. Begin raising your right hand up to chest height.

9 Turn your left toe inward, making your left leg straighten and stretch fully. Continue raising your right hand to chest level and drop your left arm while opening and twisting the hand.

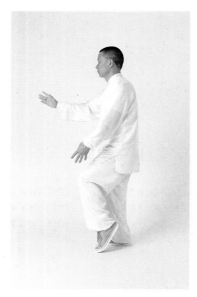

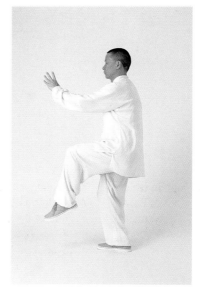

10 Exhaling, step forward with your left foot. Begin dropping your right hand and sweeping forward your now unhooked left hand.

11 Finish by raising your left leg while keeping the right leg bent slightly at the knee. Bring your left hand up to shoulder level.

Form 18
"WORK AT SHUTTLES ON BOTH SIDES"

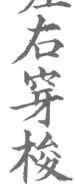

左右穿梭

This Form reflects the actively defensive nature of *Tai Chi*, using the sweeping movement of the arms to protect the head from a supposed opponent. To create the "shuttles," push the hands out to attack the opponent's face, while keeping yourself within a protective cocoon. Always time your hands to match your steps.

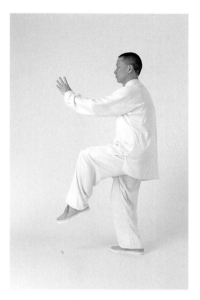

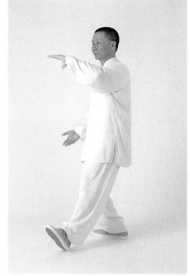

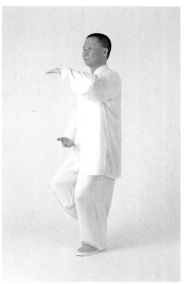

1 Begin in the position in which you ended the previous Form —with your left leg raised, right leg bent, and left hand up at shoulder level.

2 Inhaling, make a half turn to the left as you place your left foot on the ground, heel first, ahead and to the left of your right foot.

3 Shift your weight forward onto your left foot, bringing your right foot up beside it, while moving your arms into a "hold-ball" position (see page 28).

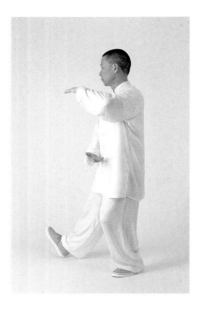

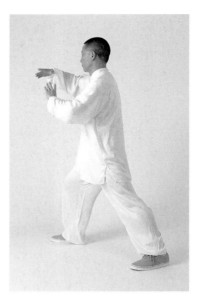

4 Turning to the right, step out with your right foot, heel first, looking in the direction of your step.

5 Exhaling, swing your right arm up and out, rotating the hand to palm down. Turn the left hand palm outward as it pushes forward. Start to shift forward your weight.

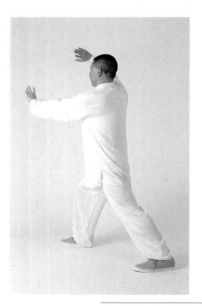

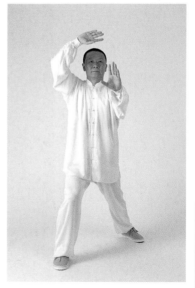

6 Lean forward into a right-footed bow stance (see page 31), bringing your right hand up above your head and pushing out with your left to make a frame with your arms (see alternative view, right).

From the front, you can see how you should be looking straight ahead through the frame made by your arms.

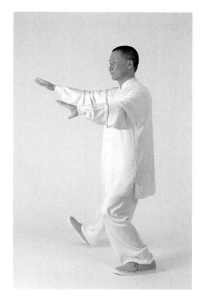

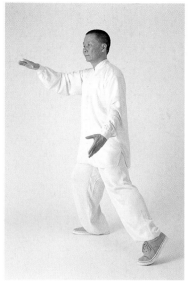

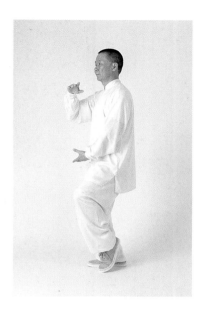

7 Inhaling, bring both hands downward, palms facing toward the ground, lean backward over your bent left leg using your right heel as a pivot, and turn to the left.

8 Lean to the right and begin stepping over with your left leg, while making an arc with your left arm down and across your waist, and moving your right arm toward your body.

9 Step across into a left-footed empty step (see page 33) as your hands come into a "hold-ball" position, with the right hand uppermost.

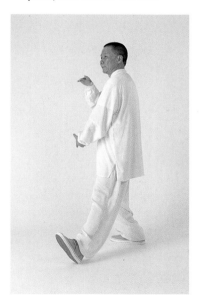

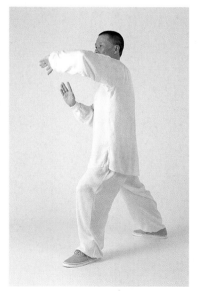

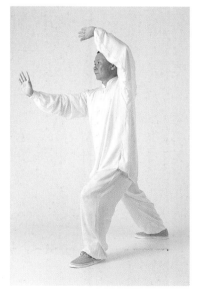

10 Repeat the movement in reverse by stepping out with your left leg, heel first.

11 Exhaling, step forward into a left-footed bow stance, bringing your left arm up above shoulder height and pushing out with your right hand, all the time keeping your body upright.

12 Finish with your right hand thrust forward and your left arm above your head.

Form 19

"NEEDLE AT THE BOTTOM OF THE SEA"

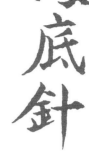

The downward thrust of the right hand in this Form should gain its power from the waist. The power is then transferred all the way through the back and right shoulder and elbow to the fingers. By focusing on the *dan tian* (see page 30) and keeping the movement compact, you can utilize a huge amount of energy in this Form.

HINTS & TIPS

• While working through this Form, turn your body at the waist as you step first one way then the other.

• The waist leads the arms, hands, legs, and feet.

• When the left leg bends forward, let it take all your body weight.

• In the final movement, keep the back and neck straight, bend only at the waist.

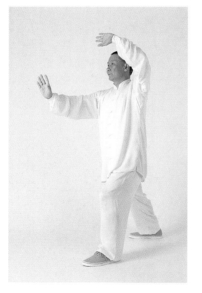

1 Begin in the position in which you ended the previous Form —in a left-footed bow stance (see page 31) with your right hand thrust forward and your left arm above head height.

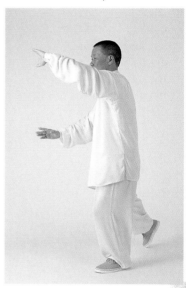

2 Breathing in, move your body forward taking the weight on your left leg, knee slightly bent, and lower both hands, palms downward.

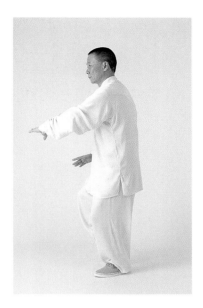

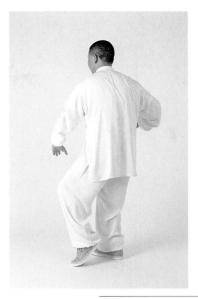

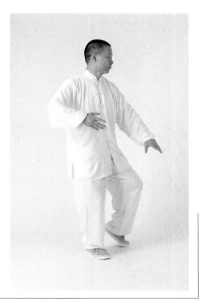

3 Step up out of the left-footed bow stance by bringing your right foot forward alongside your left as your hands reach waist height.

4 Turn to the right as you shift your weight onto your right foot and lift up your left heel (see alternative view, right).

As you shift your weight from one foot to the other, keep both elbows in close beside your body.

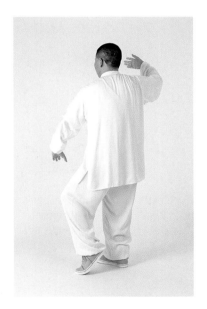

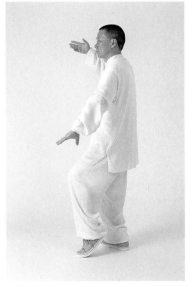

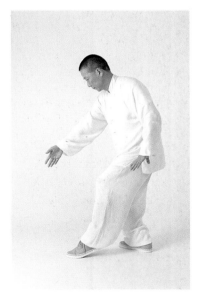

5 Exhaling, keep your feet in the same position as you turn from the waist toward the right, while bringing your right hand back up to eye level.

6 Turn your body back to the left. Begin to swing your right arm back down in front of your body. Aim your hand at an imaginary point in front of you.

7 Bending at the waist, thrust your right hand down from the shoulder. Keep your left hand, palm down, by your hip. Step your left leg forward until your toes touch down. Look along your fingers at the ground.

Form 20

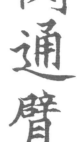

"FLASH ARM"

Ensure that all your movements curve smoothly through the air and stretch your arms fully. Try to feel fully grounded during this Form—like a tree whose roots are bound into the earth. As you open your arms for the bow stance (see page 31), imagine that you have the strength to hold up the sky.

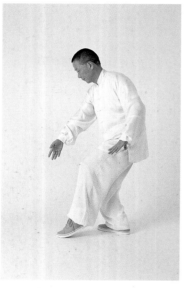  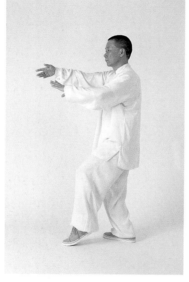 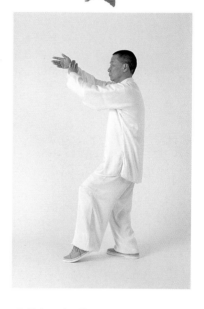

1 Begin in the position in which you ended the previous Form—with both knees bent in a left-footed empty step (see page 33), with your right hand pointing downward, and your left hand by your hip, palm down.

2 Inhaling, stand up straight, rising from the waist and keeping your left foot in the empty step. Form an arc with both your arms, elbows bent, around your chest.

3 Bring the fingers of your left hand up to rest on the wrist of your right hand.

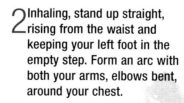

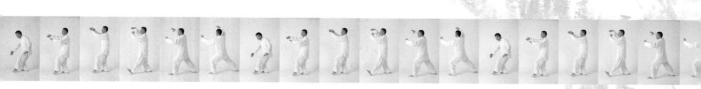

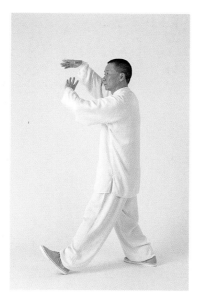

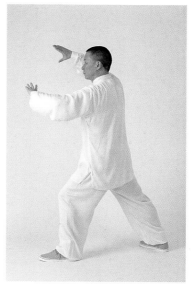

4 Pivot your left leg using the heel of your left foot, while moving both hands apart.

5 Exhaling, move forward into a left-footed bow stance (see page 31), turning slightly to the right. Push your left hand away from your face. Start turning the right palm out.

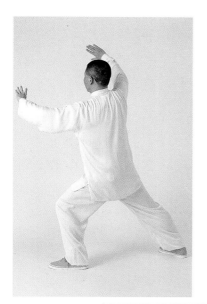

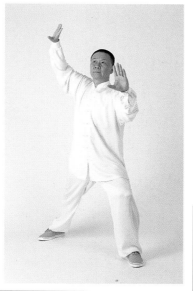

6 Exhaling, finish in a full bow stance with your arms spread. Gaze at your left hand (see alternative view, right).

When moving forward into the bow stance, turn slightly to the right. As you push your left hand away from your face ensure that it in line with your other hand.

HINTS & TIPS

• Expansive sweeping with your arms opens out your chest and naturally results in an open bow stance.

• During the left-footed bow stance, push the left knee forward at the same time as the left hand pushes forward, and the right hand pushes upward.

Form 21

"TURN DOWNWARD TO DEFLECT, PARRY, AND PUNCH"

Step with cat-like movements, and keep your fist hollow as you punch straight out. This Form is based on the action of defending from an attacker by turning, parrying, and retaliating. Coordinating the different elements will help your balance and control.

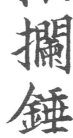

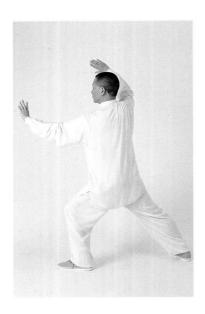

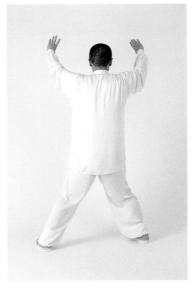

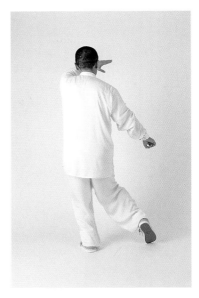

1 Begin in the position in which you ended the previous Form —in a full bow stance with arms spread, right hand above your forehead, left hand at shoulder height.

2 Inhaling, sit back, shifting your weight onto your right leg, turning your body to the right and the toes of your left foot inward while raising both hands above eye level, palms outward.

3 Shift your weight back to the left and raise your right heel. At the same time arc your right arm down, with your hand in a fist (see page 26). Bring your left hand in front of your eyes, palm facing downward.

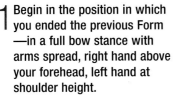

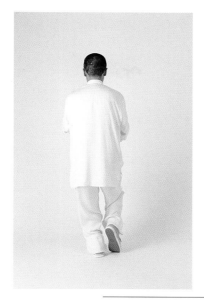

4 Move your right foot beside your left, and your right-hand fist up into your chest behind your open-palmed left hand (see alternative view, right).

Hide your fist behind the downward-facing, left palm.

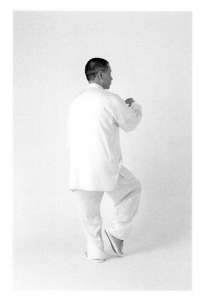

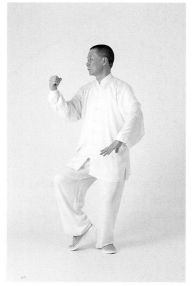

5 Exhaling, turn to the right, with your right fist continuing to move upward (see alternative view, right).

The right fist moves upward to chin height. Also bring your left arm downward, palm pressing toward the floor.

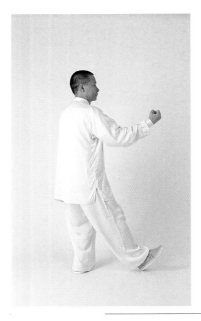

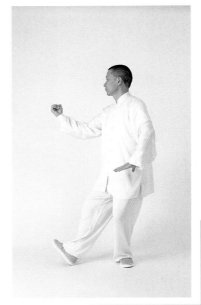

6 Step out with your right foot, heel down first. Bring your fist out in a backhand punch and lower your left hand beside your hip, palm down.

This view shows the left hand held palm down beside your hip as you step forward. The fingers of the right hand are curled toward you.

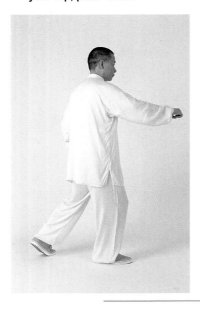

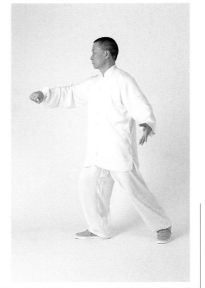

7 Inhaling, move forward by placing your right foot fully on the floor. Turn both hands to the left (see alternative view, right). Step around your right foot with your left.

By the end of the punch, both wrists should have completed their left turns so that ultimately they face downward.

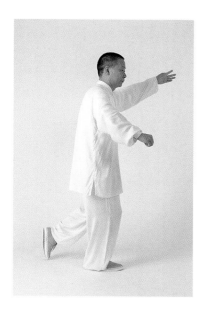

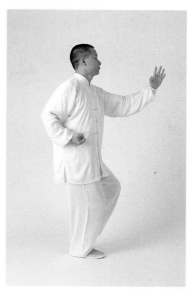

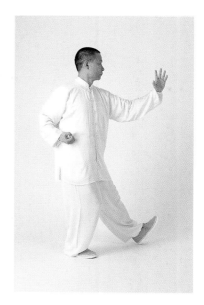

8 Move forward, raising your left arm past eye level while pulling your right fist backward.

9 Hold your right fist by your waist, fingers curled up, and your left arm out ahead of you, elbow bent ready to punch forward.

10 Move the left foot out, heel to the ground, in preparation for the next punch.

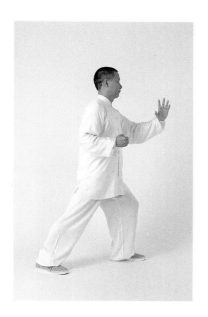

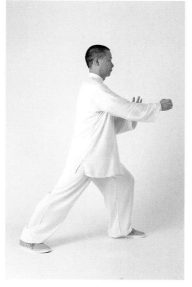

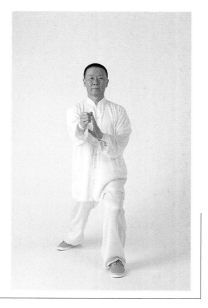

11 Bring your body weight forward onto your left leg as you start the punch.

12 Step into a left-footed bow stance (see page 31) as you punch out with your right hand, bringing your left hand back when you reach full stretch (see alternative view, right).

Bring your left hand alongside the right arm as you finish the movement.

Form 22

"APPARENT CLOSE-UP"

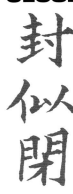

When the body moves, the torso should remain upright and straight, especially when standing in the bow stance (see page 31). The body should hardly turn in this Form. Give complete concentration to the lifting of the arms and the slight movement of the body backward and forward.

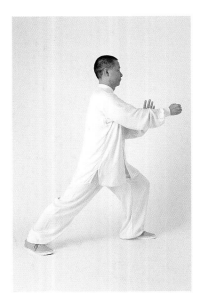

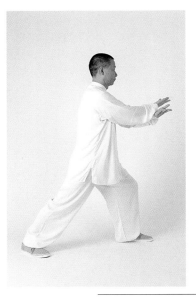

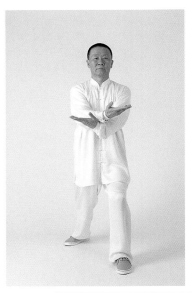

1 Begin in the position in which you ended the previous Form —in a left-footed bow stance (see page 31) with your right fist punching at full stretch, and the left arm alongside the right arm.

2 Unclench your right hand and, inhaling, move the left hand forward bringing it underneath and past your right hand (see right). Both hands should have palms upwards.

From the front, you can see that the arms cross at the wrist, the right arm uppermost.

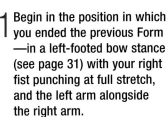

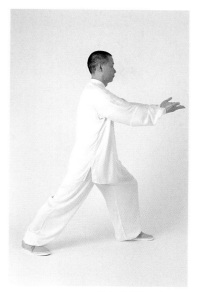

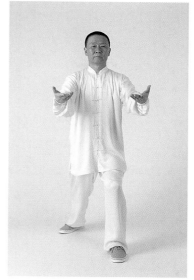

3 Keep your arms outstretched and uncross your wrists (see alternative view, right).

As you uncross your wrists, ensure that your hands do not swing beyond the sides of your body.

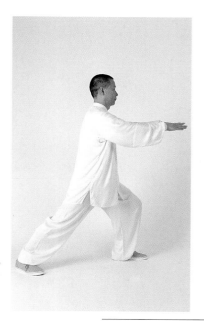

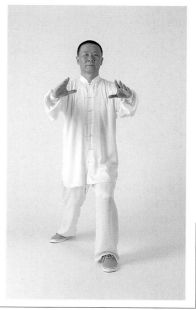

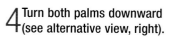

4 Turn both palms downward (see alternative view, right).

Again, the hands should stay within the width of the sides of your body. Take care not to swing your arms outward as you turn your hands over.

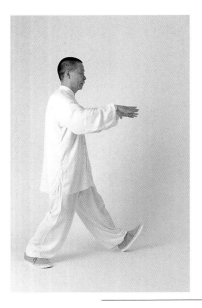

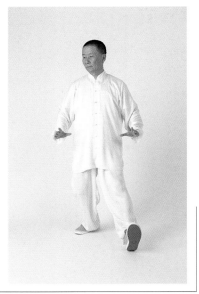

5 Moving back out of the bow stance, shift your weight onto your right leg, rocking on your left heel. Bring your hands back toward your chest.

Seen from in front, you can see that you should look to the right as you move back and turn your palms downward.

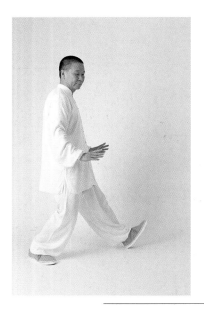

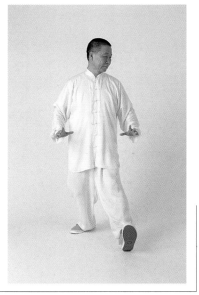

6 Lower your hands, and as you drop them in front of your stomach, bend your right knee, ready for the final push.

Hold the position as you turn to look to the left.

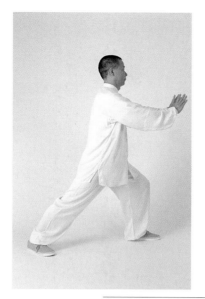

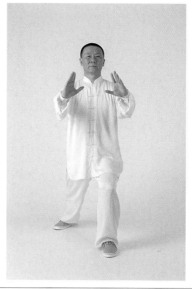

7 Exhaling, look straight ahead and move forward into a left-footed bow stance, pushing your hands up and out in front of you (see alternative view, right).

As you hold your palms outward in front of you, ensure that they are at chest height.

HINTS & TIPS

• Try to stay within your own body's space. This will create a protective shell around you, from which you can push out.

• Hold your elbows directly below your shoulders and keep your shoulders relaxed.

• When pushing out with your hands, let your energy flow up through your feet, which should still be rooted to the ground. Channel the force through the *dan tian* (see page 30), to give you maximum mental energy: as the Chinese say, the power "to push over a mountain or a ship into harbor."

• Lead all movements from the waist.

Form 23

"CROSS HANDS"

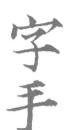

十
字
手

Keep your hands moving in smooth circles, whatever your body is doing. Think of the working of a clock: the movement of the hands is regular and continuous, even though the cogs of the mechanism are of different sizes and move at different speeds and in different directions. In this Form, your hands are like the hands of the clock.

HINTS & TIPS

• Sweep your arms moving in smooth, continuous circles throughout your body's shifts of weight and changes in direction.

• Keep your head still and level—don't let yourself bounce up and down.

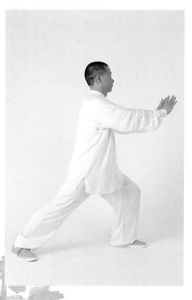

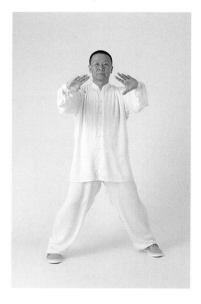

1 Begin in the position in which you ended the previous Form—in a left-footed bow stance, pushing your hands up and out in front of you.

2 Inhaling, bend your right knee, sit back and turn 90° to the right. Turn your left toe inward but keep your hands in front of you.

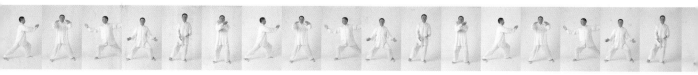

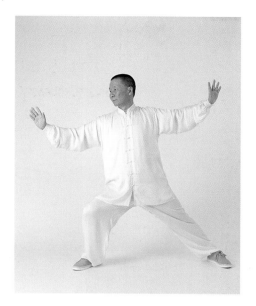

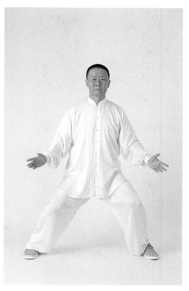

3 Open out your arms and shift your weight to the right, all the time watching your right hand.

4 Slowly shift your weight back leftward to center your body in a riding-horse stance (see page 32) while moving your hands downward.

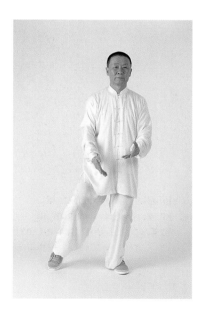

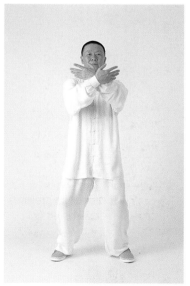

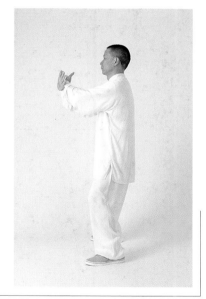

5 Gradually move your weight left, lifting your right heel as you do so, and moving your hands inward.

6 Finish with your knees slightly bent and your wrists crossed in front of the top of your chest (see alternative view, right).

From this angle, you can see that you should hold your hands well out from your body.

Form 24

"CLOSING FORM"

Relax but try not to be loose as you hold this Form. Breathe deeply and naturally. Although you may seem to be moving very little, you will find that this Form is one of the most important because of the way it calms the brain. Be methodical in perfecting the simple steps.

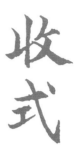

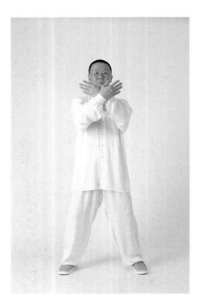

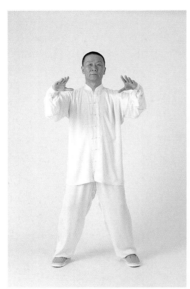

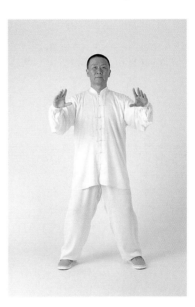

1 Begin in the position in which you ended the previous Form —with your knees slightly bent and your wrists crossed in front of you at the top of your chest.

2 Breathing in, open your hands, turning your palms downward.

3 Breathing out, press downward with your elbows leading the hands.

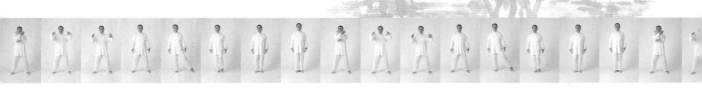

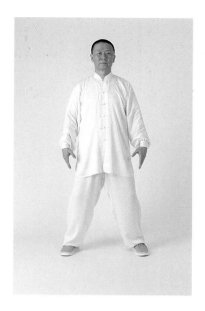

4 Turn your palms in as you lower your arms to your sides.

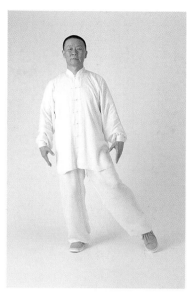

5 Shift your weight onto your right foot and lift up your left heel.

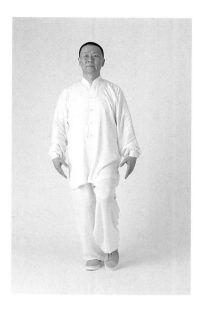

6 Bring your left foot in, placing your left toes beside the right foot.

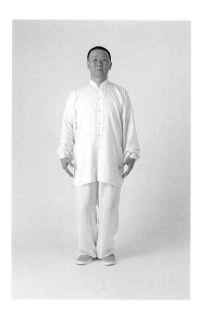

7 Lower your left heel and let your heels touch and your toes open with your weight centered.

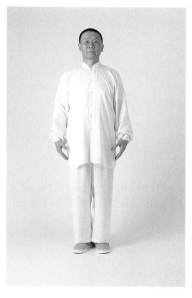

8 Standing upright, look straight ahead and take a deep breath.

HINTS & TIPS

• Stretch up from the very top of your head, pushing your chin in.

• Hold your chest in, straighten your spine, and relax your shoulders.

• Hold your tummy in and concentrate on your *dan tian* (see page 30).

• Let your mind empty.

Eye Exercises

The health of the eyes is vital to our general wellbeing throughout our life. As we age, they can become a source of problems so it is vital to protect their health as much as possible. Like any other part of the body, the eyes need exercise, and this has never been more important than today with the rapid growth in the use of televisions and computer displays. The exercises that follow relax the muscles that can become stiff and tired if the eyes focus for any length of time on a screen. Pressing the acupressure points along the channels at the back of the neck and on the hands also relate directly to the good health of the eyes.

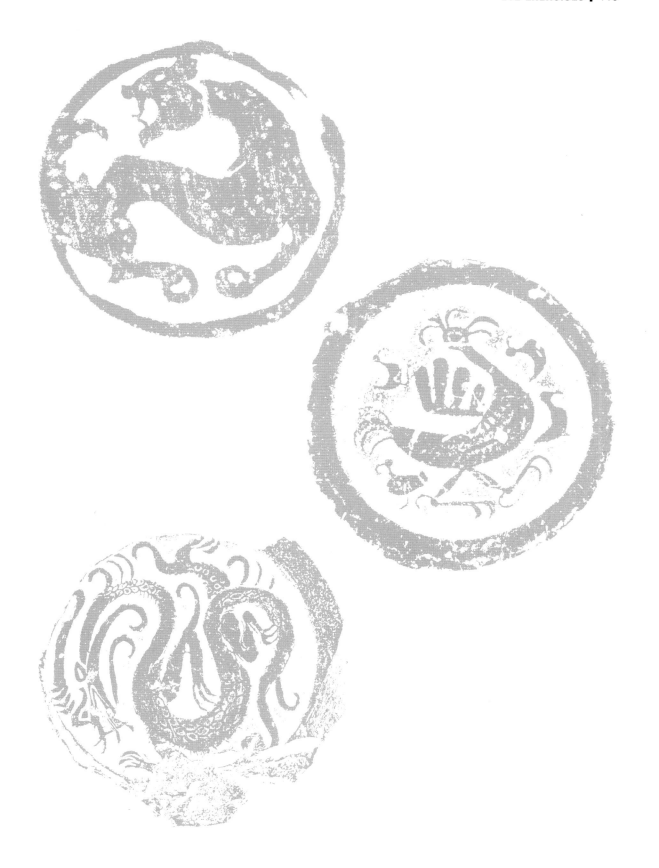

Introduction

Work around the eyes, massaging the acupressure points that are related to them. Use the index, middle, or both fingers, depending on the amount of pressure you wish to exert. Use just enough pressure to give an aching, swollen feeling—this is a sure sign that the massage is doing its job.

Relax your entire body, breathing normally. For each of the first eight exercises, find the relevant pressure point, as marked below or on the hand in the eighth exercise (*He Gu*), and slowly make circles around the spot, counting to 8 first in one direction, then the other, before repeating the whole exercise.

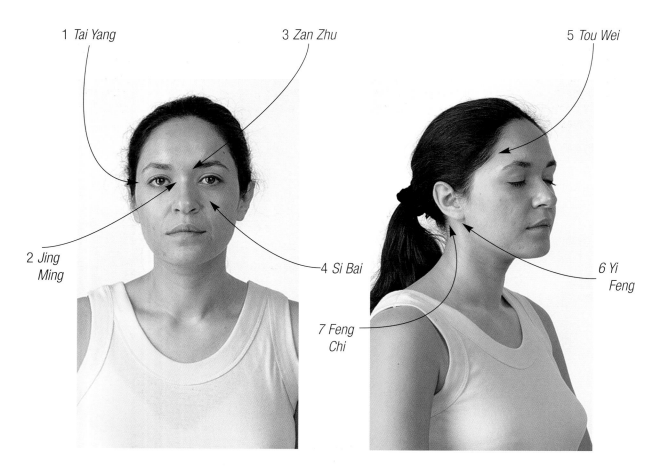

1 *Tai Yang*

3 *Zan Zhu*

5 *Tou Wei*

2 *Jing Ming*

4 *Si Bai*

6 *Yi Feng*

7 *Feng Chi*

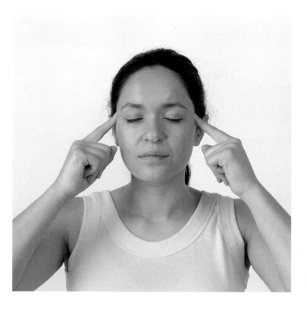

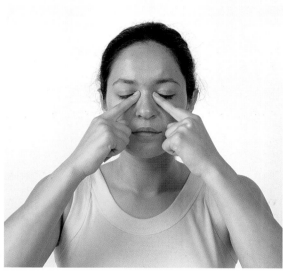

Exercise 1—*Tai Yang*
Relax, close your eyes, and begin massaging the first of the acupressure points about an inch beside the eyes. Place your fingers in line with the center of your eyes in the middle of your temples. Rotate slowly forward and back, counting to eight each time, then repeat.

Exercise 2—*Jing Ming*
Move your fingers to each side of your nose, just by the inner points of your eyes. You may want to use a different amount of pressure here—you want to use enough pressure to create the same aching feeling of the first exercise.

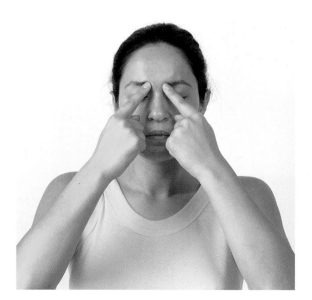

Exercise 3—*Zan Zhu*
The third point is just above the eyes on the edge of the brow. Press up into the brow from below, either side of the bridge of your nose. Stay relaxed, with your eyes naturally closed, and breath normally throughout.

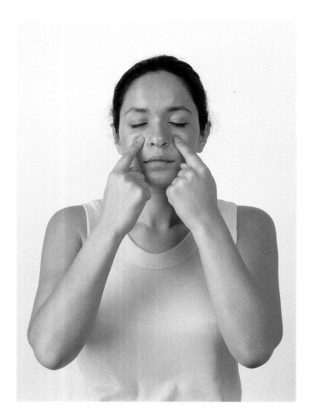

Exercise 4—*Si Bai*

Move down to the fourth pressure point, situated at the top of the cheekbone about an inch under the center of both eyes. To find the spot, run your fingers down your cheek from the center of each eye until they cross the top ridge of your cheekbone and massage the hollow area just below, in line with the flaring of your nostrils.

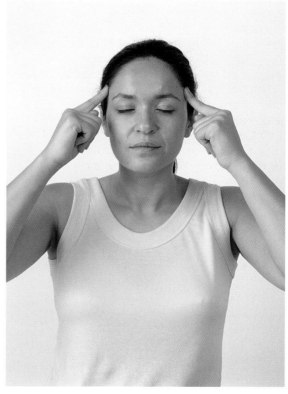

Exercise 5—*Tou Wei*

Move your fingers back up to your temples to find the second pressure point on the side of the face. This time, the pressure point is above the eye, almost on the hairline, underneath the muscles that flex when you bite your teeth. You may want to use slightly more pressure here to achieve a similar sensation.

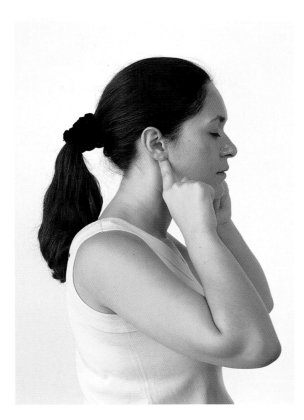

Exercise 6—*Yi Feng*

The 12 channels running through the body that are used in both Chinese medicine and acupuncture have points along them that relate to organs situated some distance away. Two points around the base of the ear relate directly to the eyes. The first—directly below the ear between the jawbone and the tendon running down the neck—can be found by resting your first finger along the back of your jaw and pressing behind the earlobe.

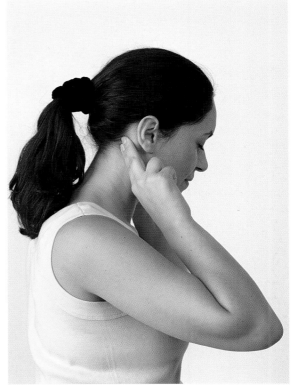

Exercise 7—*Feng Chi*

The second acupressure point behind the ear is on the same level as the first but further round to the back, against the edge of the cranium. Find it by moving your fingers back over the tendons to the hairline and press up underneath the bottom of the skull.

Exercise 8—*He Gu*

The channel running from fingertips to shoulder includes a spot between the thumb and first finger that is the final, single pressure point for protecting the eyes. Be careful not to apply too much pressure—this is a very sensitive spot and you are using your thumb for the first time.

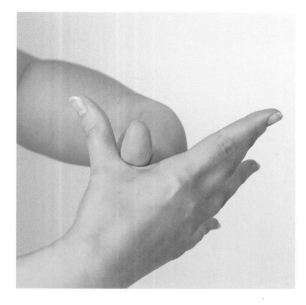

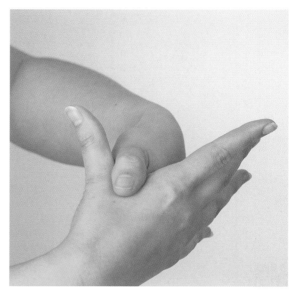

1 Find the pressure point by opening out the thumb and first finger of your right hand and placing the top joint of your other thumb against the flap of skin between the two digits.

2 Resting your right hand on the left-hand first finger of your left hand, drop your left thumb down to rest between the thumb and first finger.

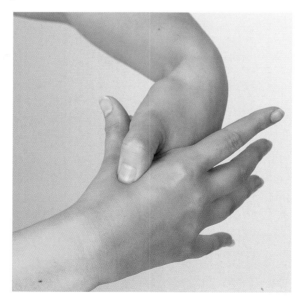

3 Press down with the tip of your left thumb and rotate in both directions twice.

Exercise 9—The First *Lu*

Massaging the eyebrows and sides of your face brings various points together in a single movement. This first exercise smoothes out the points above and to the sides of the eye with the fingers. Use the sides of your first fingers and, once again, press as hard as is appropriate to achieve a dull, but therapeutic aching sensation.

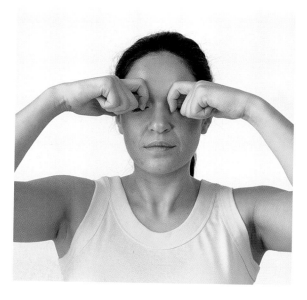

1 Place your thumbs, pointing backwards, across your temples and rest your curved first fingers along your brow, encircling your eyebrows, over the pressure point massaged in Exercise 3.

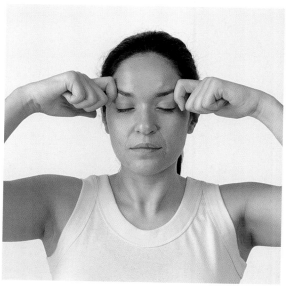

2 Using the middle section of your first finger, rub your brow line, lifting your thumbs away from the side of your face as you progress.

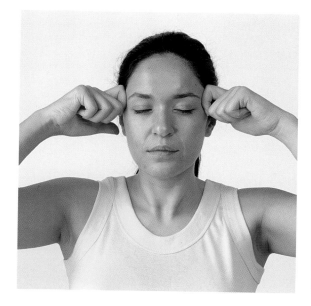

3 Pull your fingers across your temples, over and beyond the pressure point massaged in Exercise 1.

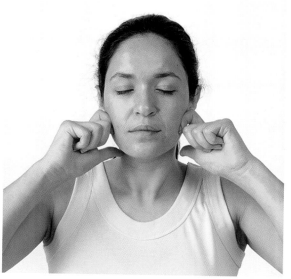

4 Pull your fingers down the sides of your face, gently releasing the pressure as you move past your ears. Repeat the exercise three times.

Exercise 10—The Second *Lu*

This exercise combines the pressure points down the front of your face. Although you are using only the tips of your first fingers, you can use just as much pressure as in the previous exercise. By moving down the face, you are incorporating separate points on the same channel, uniting them in a single movement.

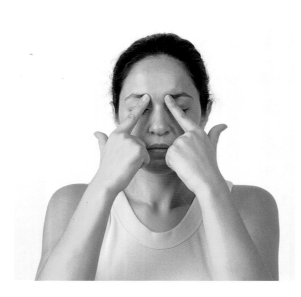

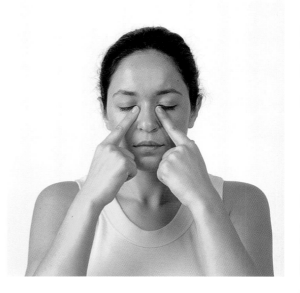

1 Start by holding the tips of your fingers against the pressure point on the edge of your brow.

2 Pull your fingers slowly downwards along the side of your nose over the point massaged in Exercise 2.

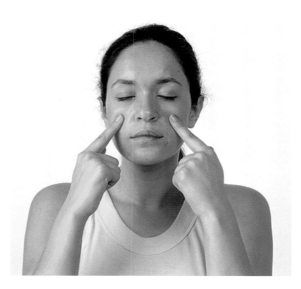

3 Continue down your cheeks, covering the points massaged in Exercise 4 before releasing the pressure. Repeat the exercise three times.

Exercise 11—*Jing Mo, An Shi,* and *Yuan Tiao*

Finish by allowing your eyes to relax completely, letting the muscles that hold your eyes in focus to go loose. Combining this meditative relaxation with the previous exercises should help your eyes stay stronger for longer.

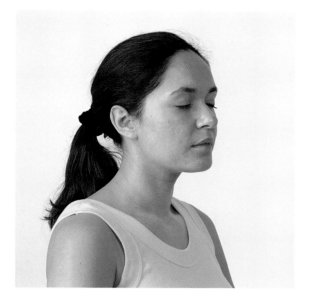

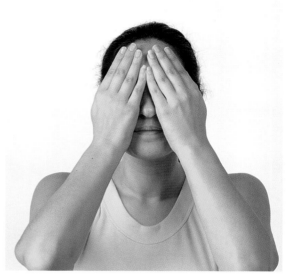

1 Close your eyes and relax your whole body, naturally deeply breathing, letting every muscle go loose, thinking especially of your eyes. Let them settle into a state of gentle stillness, or *Jing Mo*.

2 Now, during *An Shi*, block out all light with your hands and open your eyes, looking as far into the black distance as possible. The more relaxed your eye muscles, the further you will seem to look.

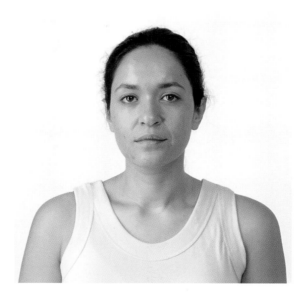

3 When you feel completely relaxed, move into *Yuan Tiao*. Open your eyes but don't let them focus: stare into the far distance until you are ready to finish.

Index